Health and Social Class in Imperial Germany
A Social History of Mortality, Morbidity and Inequality

REINHARD SPREE

Health and Social Class in Imperial Germany
A Social History of Mortality, Morbidity and Inequality

With a Foreword by
PAUL WEINDLING

Translated from the German by
STUART MCKINNON-EVANS (MATERIAL WORD)
in association with JOHN HALLIDAY

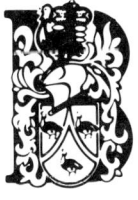

BERG
Oxford / New York / Hamburg

Distributed exclusively in the US and Canada by
St. Martin's Press, New York

First published in 1988 by
Berg Publishers Limited
Market House, Deddington, Oxford OX5 4SW, UK
175 Fifth Avenue/Room 400, New York, NY 10010, USA
Schenefelder Landstr. 14K, 2000 Hamburg 55, FRG

Originally published as *Soziale Ungleichheit vor Krankheit und Tod. Zur Sozialgeschichte des Gesundheitsbereichs im Deutschen Kaiserreich.* Translated from the German by permission of the publishers, Vandenhoeck & Ruprecht, Göttingen. © Vandenhoeck & Ruprecht in Göttingen 1981
English translation © Berg Publishers Limited 1988

All rights reserved

British Library Cataloguing in Publication Data

Spree, Reinhard
  Health and social class in Imperial
  Germany: a social history of mortality,
  morbidity and inequality.
  1. Medical care—Social aspects—
  Germany   2. Medical care—Germany—
  History
  I. Title II. Soziale Ungleichheit vor
  Krankheit und Tod. *English*
  362.1′0943   RA395.G3

  ISBN 0–85496–527–0

Library of Congress Cataloging-in-Publication Data

Spree, Reinhard.
  Health and social class in Imperial Germany.
  Translation of: Soziale Ungleichheit vor Krankheit und Tod.
    Bibliography: p.
    Includes index.
    1. Social medicine—Germany—History. 2. Social classes—Germany—History. 3. Mortality—Social aspects—Germany—History. I. Title.
  RA418.3.G3S6713 1988   362.1′0943   87–22397
  ISBN 0–85496–527–0

Printed in Great Britain by Billings of Worcester

Contents

Foreword *Paul Weindling* — 1

Preface — 5

Introduction: A Theoretical Framework for the Impact of Class Formation and Stratification on Chances of Survival — 11

Part I Changes in Health and Mortality — 21

1. Changes in the 'People's Health' — 23
   1.1. Different Approaches 23
   1.2. Basic Concepts, Problems of Measurement and Sources 26
   1.3. Changes in Mortality Rates and the Course of the 'People's Health' 35
   1.4. Changes in the Pattern of Causes of Death 40
   1.5. Summary: Changing Trends in the 'People's Health' 47

2. Infant Mortality as a Mirror of Social Inequality — 55
   2.1. Infant Mortality as an Indicator: Concepts and Sources 55
   2.2. Infant Mortality and Parental Wealth 60
   2.3. Infant Mortality and Parental Occupation 63
   2.4. Infant Mortality and Diet 71
   2.5. Recapitulation 80
   2.6. Infant Mortality and Birth Control 84
   2.7. Hypotheses on the Interrelation between Market Capacity and Family Planning 95

Part II Determinants of the Decline in Mortality — 103

3. The Expansion of the Health Sector — 109
   3.1. Evidence of Quantitative Changes 110
   3.2. Changes in the Quality of Care 116
   3.3. The Relationship between the Expansion of the Health Sector and the Decline in Mortality 121

4.	The Expansion of the Health-related Infrastructure	131
	4.1. Drinking-water Supplies and Sewerage Systems 133	
	4.2. Case Study: Berlin 139	
	4.3. Summary 144	
5.	Changes in Income and Diet	145
6.	Summary	150

Part III The Medicalisation of the Population, the Professionalisation of Doctors and Socio-structural Change   155

7.	A Theoretical Framework for an Analysis of Professionalisation	157
8.	Medical Reforms and the Suppression of Lay Healers in the Mid-Nineteenth Century	160
9.	Integration of Competing Interests, Resistance to Social Regulation, and Professionalisation	166
10.	Resistance to Monopolisation of the Medical Market by Doctors	171
11.	'Enforced Socialisation' of the Lower Classes and Medicalisation	178

Conclusion   185

Appendix: Tables 1–25   189

Bibliography   222

Index   241

Tables

1. Mortality rates in various age groups and regions in Prussia in 1876, 1901 and 1913 — 191
2. Mortality rates in various age groups in 22 large Prussian towns and in Prussia as a whole in 1876 and 1900 — 192
3. Correlation between infant mortality rate and welfare, and excess mortality rates in urban districts of Berlin from 1886 to 1910 — 193
4. Infant mortality rates in different occupational groups in Prussia from 1877 to 1913 — 194
5. Excess infant mortality rates in different occupational groups in Prussia from 1877 to 1913 — 195
6. Infant mortality rates in different occupational groups in Prussia from 1902 to 1913 — 196
7. Percentage of legitimate infants breast-fed in various income groups in selected towns and rural districts of western Germany from 1905 to 1911 — 197
8. Breast-feeding and mortality of legitimate infants in various income groups in the administrative district of Düsseldorf from 1905 to 1911 — 198
9. Breast-feeding and mortality of legitimate infants in various income groups in Hanover and Linden in 1911–12 — 198
10. Breast-feeding, legitimacy and mother's employment in Hanover in 1912 — 199
11. Duration of breast-feeding of legitimate infants in selected areas of north-west Germany in different income groups from 1905 to 1912 — 201
12. Duration of breast-feeding of legitimate infants living with their mothers on 4 June 1912 in Hanover, in different occupational groups — 202
13. Average number of children per complete marriage in various social groups in Lower Saxony from the end of the eighteenth century to 1914 — 203
14. Average number of children per marriage in the

German Reich, by occupation, economic sector and year of marriage	204
15. Average number of children per marriage in the non-agricultural population of the German Reich, by occupation, size of community and year of marriage	205
16. Average number of children per marriage in the German Reich, late-nineteenth and early-twentieth centuries, by 43 occupations and year of marriage	206
17. Distribution of married couples in each occupational group by number of children and year of marriage	209
18. Regional distribution of doctors and members of statutory sickness insurance funds in the German Reich in 1885–7 and 1907–9	214
19. Distribution of 'quacks' in Prussian administrative districts and their ratio to doctors in 1903 and 1913	215
20. Members of statutory sickness insurance funds in the German Reich, 1885–1911	216
21. Number of hospital patients and mortality in Prussian administrative districts, 1880 and 1913	217
22. Central water supply systems in German towns of at least 2000 inhabitants *circa* 1895: comparison by size	218
23. Percentage of population of Prussian administrative districts resident in places with central water supply systems in 1900	219
24. Increase in number of towns in the German Reich with central water supply systems from 1870 to 1900	220
25. Average mortality rates in relation to wealth and hygiene conditions in urban districts of Berlin, 1875 and 1890	221

Figure

1. Infant mortality among various occupational groups in Prussia, 1877–1914	65

Foreword

Deaths and diseases provide sensitive indicators of the social impact of such crucial social changes as industrialisation and the transition to smaller families. How economic and social upheavals affect different social groups is an issue that social scientists and historians can help to clarify. Studies of inequalities in health are a means of examining crucial processes of social change. These issues raise a combination of economic, cultural and political questions. How economic differentials affect the market for medical care, and how this market itself structures the organisation and professional institutions of the providers of care are problems that have only begun to gain attention. Historical and comparative studies are fundamental to understanding how patterns of inequality undergo structural changes over long periods. Reinhard Spree's study is to be welcomed as an innovative and perceptive case study of changing patterns of social inequality at a crucial period of German and European history.

Today's major issues in health care need understanding in a broader social, political and historical context. The social historian has a strong sense of *déjà vu* with regard to current concerns over social inequalities in health, the links between unemployment and sickness, and (as a result of concern with cancer, heart disease and lately AIDS) medicine as a way of promoting changes in life style. All these problems require analysis not only in scientific and epidemiological terms, but also by applying the methods and categories of social science. Life expectancy, the prevalence of chronic ill-health and access to medical services are all affected by economic factors related to occupation, social status and gender. The 1980 *Black Report* on inequalities in health took the differential experiences of occupational classes as its starting point.[1] It is sobering that in a modern welfare state with — in theory — equal access to health services that 'at birth and during the first month of life the risk of death in families of unskilled workers is double that of professional families'. The poorer health experience of lower-

---

1. P. Townsend and N. Davidson (eds), *Inequalities in Health. The Black Report*, Harmondsworth, 1982.

occupational groups applies at all stages of life. That economic deprivation is compounded by worse health, shorter life expectancy, and higher rates of disease and death among dependants is a familiar feature to social historians.

The case of Imperial Germany is well worth the attention of social scientists. It experienced rates of industrialisation, urban expansion and population growth which were the most rapid in nineteenth-century Europe. There resulted a modern and highly innovative economy. Although the pace of change was uneven, rural populations were also affected by changing patterns of labour and in birth rates that influenced health. The human impact of industrialisation can be gauged in terms of mass social deprivation reflected in housing shortage, low incomes and the first experience for many of the faster pace and higher risks of industrial working conditions. Other effects of industrialisation were similarly striking: demographically, the decline in the birth rate — a process first evident among the professional and bureaucratic classes — was especially pronounced; and the political tensions with the rise of a mass socialist party confronting a Junker and militarily dominated state were immense. At the same time Germany evolved one of the most innovative systems of training medical researchers and doctors. The introduction of sickness insurance in 1883 was a breakthrough in the social sphere that has been emulated throughout the world. By 1900 the German medical profession not only led the world in terms of its scientific training, but also in its militancy in defending its economic interests. Given the emerging power of the economy and the politically destabilising results of unresolved tensions in German society, the experience of social change in Germany has immense importance.

Spree's work is innovative in that he examines differentials in German society in terms that go beyond strictly economic categories. He considers differentials in health from the point of view of social stratification. He thus is able to examine processes that affected not only general considerations of social policy, but the everyday lives of the population. The closest comparison to his work for nineteenth-century Britain is F.B. Smith's evocative analysis of *The People's Health* by means of the differential experience of age groups.[2] Like Spree, Smith's analysis contributes to a new social history of medicine concerned with the health of populations rather than with innovations in medical science. Yet Spree's work is characterised by greater attention to the statistics produced

---

2. F.B. Smith, *The People's Health. 1830–1910*, London, 1979.

by states, municipalities and sickness insurance providers, as well as by a sophisticated analysis of the relations between class, occupation and the economy. The statistics of social differentials make it possible to judge how widely applicable more qualitative developments were.

Spree's starting-point is the Weberian analysis of the relations between class and the expanding market economy. Differentials in mortality are related to the distribution of wealth, but — following the Weberian distinction between class and *Stand* or social status group — distinctive values associated with the *Stand* are also important. These include eating habits, clothing, social customs and attitudes to health and disease. In contrast to demographers seeing changes in mentality as due to life expectancy, Spree regards the incidence of death and disease as actively affecting the process of class formation by a causal nexus between the *Stand* and class. Economic factors are also extended into the sphere of medicine. Spree is innovative in applying the concept of a market demand for health care. This is valuable in raising the issues of popular attitudes to health and of doctor–patient relations that are central to the social history of medicine.

This work is a major innovation in the use of health issues to analyse social structure. It opens the way to further investigations not just of mortality rates, but also of chronic diseases such as TB. These had a high incidence in areas of social deprivation, and are revealing of poverty, poor housing and malnutrition, as well as of prevailing ideologies, professional attitudes and social structure. Infant diseases were important, as their incidence was — and is — a generally accepted index of health in developing societies. Spree relates infant health to economic factors, such as women's work, as well as to changing attitudes towards the family. Sickness insurance is another area of great potential for the study of morbidity in relation to social inequality. Spree examines its role as a mechanism of socialisation and as creating a state-directed widening market for medical care.

Spree has been pioneering in application of economic and demographic categories to issues of health, disease and associated issues of professionalisation. He has encouraged and co-operated in a new wave of research by German social scientists on the social history of medicine.[3] Substantial studies by social historians of such topics as

---

3. A. Labisch, R. Spree and P.J. Weindling, 'Social History of Nineteenth and Twentieth Century German Medicine', *Bulletin of the Society for the Social History of Medicine*, 32 (1983), pp. 40–5.

professionalisation, sickness insurance and of municipal health services have shown how health was a major political, economic and everyday concern. Such studies form substantial contributions for analysis of social and economic modernisation and social status, and of political aspects of the welfare state. These approaches draw on the generation of studies by the French *Annales* school of historians on the mentalities associated with birth, marriage and death, as well as on studies by British social historians of social protest and political mobilisation.[4]

The new German work on the social history of medicine should be regarded as innovative in its own right, in such areas as the study of sickness insurance, as well as regarding such concepts as the rationalisation of life style in response to industrialisation. The new wave of German social history of medicine raises the challenging issue as to whether medicine affects life style more through such agencies of 'compulsory socialisation' as sickness insurance, or through an informal 'civilising process'. Certainly English-language readers will be struck by many features that are characteristic of the German experience of industrialisation. Here, one should bear in mind that the specificity of this experience is itself a topic of major debate among social historians. Yet outweighing such discussions of the German *Sonderweg* to modernity are general questions such as the relation of earning capacity and social status to health. It is because of the relevance of these issues to the persistent inequalities in health in advanced societies that this book deserves the attention of the English-language reader.

Paul Weindling
University of Oxford
Wellcome Unit for the History of Medicine

---

4. For an extensive bibliography of work on the social history of German medicine, see P.J. Weindling, 'Medicine and Modernisation. The Social History of German Health and Medicine', *History of Science*, 24 (1986), pp. 277–301.

Preface

March 1985 saw the completion of an empirical historical study I had been conducting at the Max Planck Institute of Educational Research in Berlin. The central aim of the project was to analyse statistical data on the major groups in society in order to establish at what point around the turn of the present century 'modern' orientations, mentalities and patterns of behaviour in the sphere of familial reproduction became evident. What was particularly interesting in the study were the typical time-lags in the onset of the 'modernisation process' in various social groups.

The empirical object of investigation were the patterns of social inequality associated with the process by which young children grew up and were cared for. This process was charted and analysed using indicators based on relatively general, aggregate figures. Various dimensions of the study were identified — infant care, reproductive behaviour, levels of income and consumption. For each of these, appropriate indicators were selected, permitting a differential analysis: infant mortality rates and diet and feeding methods, the number of children per marriage and the distribution of typical family sizes, and patterns by which incomes were earned and expended. Main features of these indicators were analysed using statistics for the late nineteenth and early twentieth centuries. In order to cast light on the social context of the evidence provided by the main statistical indicators, the study was augmented by investigations into the emergence of modern health care, the health-related infrastructure, the process by which doctors became professionalised from the mid-nineteenth century onwards, and the development from the late 1700s of norms of socialisation within medicine — and particularly within paediatrics.

The purpose of the project was structured by a number of hypotheses which, on the whole, were validated. The point of departure was the assumption that social strata are not only differentiated, but are actually constituted by specific patterns of reproduction. They follow — unconsciously — what may be termed quasi-strategies that in the long term lead to uniform decisions being made in the reproductive sphere. The decision-makers are individual families, in this case mothers in particular, who determine how to acquire, distribute, expend and develop the material and immaterial resources which allow families to support themselves and pursue a particular life style. Consequently, they also make decisions about the life chances of the individual family members and their location in the social stratification system.

During the course of the 'modernisation process' in the nineteenth century, reproductive quasi-strategies were recast in a more rationalistic mould. Initially this occurred among the educated middle classes, but it gradually spread to all other social groups. The way reproduction was taking on more rationalist forms became evident first of all in spheres of everyday social activity. These were particularly susceptible to influence by individuals (and families), and they simultaneously opened up and established new life chances for groups and individuals, without being entirely dependent on the availability of material resources. Such areas of activity — family planning, the upbringing and care of children (socialisation) and consumption — form the dimensions of reproductive behaviour investigated in the project.

The indicators outlined above represent only some aspects of the dimensions of living standards and lifestyles mentioned. They point, however, to essential elements of reproductive quasi-strategies, in particular to the differences between social strata with regard to the extent to which certain features of physical and social reproduction became more rationalistic. Moreover, they clearly show the characteristic time-lags in the way this process affected the different major social groups.

The project has led to the publication of a number of articles, each of which, however, only deals with some elements of the complex subject under investigation.[1] There is a problem here,

---

1. See B. Duden and U. Ottmüller, 'Der süße Bronnen. Zur Geschichte des Stillens', *Courage*, 2 (1978), pp. 15–21; U. Ottmüller, 'Mutterschaft und romantische Liebe. Alltagsweltliche Ideologien der Familie und ihre praktischen Konsequenzen', *Sozialwissenschaftliche Informationen für Unterricht und Studium*, 8(1) (1979), pp. 12–17; idem, '"Mutterpflichten" — Die Wandlungen ihrer inhaltlichen Ausformung durch die akademische Medizin', *Gesellschaft. Beiträge zur Marxschen Theorie*, 14 (Frankfurt am Main, 1981), pp. 97–138; R. Spree, 'Strukturierte soziale Ungleichheit im Reproduktionsbereich. Zur historischen Analyse ihrer Erscheinungsformen in Deutschland 1870 bis 1913' in J. Bergmann et al. (eds), *Geschichte als politische Wissenschaft* (Stuttgart, 1979), pp. 55–115; idem, 'Die Entwicklung der differentiellen Säuglingssterblichkeit in Deutschland seit der Mitte des 19. Jahrhunderts (Ein Versuch zur Mentalitätsgeschichte)' in A.E. Imhof (ed.), *Mensch und Gesundheit in der Geschichte* (Husum, 1980), pp. 251–78; idem, 'Zur Bedeutung des Gesundheitswesens für die Entwicklung der Lebenschancen der deutschen Bevölkerung zwischen 1870 und 1913' in F. Blaich (ed.), *Staatliche Umverteilungspolitik in historischer Perspektive* (Schriften des Vereins für Socialpolitik, new series, vol. 109) (Berlin, 1980), pp. 165–223; idem, 'The Impact of the Professionalization of Physicians on Social Change in Germany during the late 19th and early 20th

Preface

because no scope is provided for portraying in sufficient detail the connections between patterns of social inequality in health, morbidity and mortality, on the one hand, and developments in health care, infrastructure and the general standard of living, on the other. This book attempts to overcome the drawbacks of a fragmentary approach by examining the range of questions involved.

The book is divided into three main parts. The introduction defines the broad context by outlining the theoretical framework adopted to describe and interpret the connection between social inequality, mortality and health, which are understood here to stand in a structured relation to one another. The framework views structures of inequality as the results of the continuous and interdependent processes of class formation and stratification. Part I describes major aspects of the dominant patterns of social inequality which relate to health and morbidity. Chapter 1 pursues the question of whether during the period under investigation the population became on average healthier as life expectancy increased, and whether any improvement in health was equally distributed among the main social groups. In Chapter 2, the social differences already outlined are quantified by using the particularly sensitive indicator of the infant mortality rate. Additional factors, which to some extent compensated for the effects of social inequalities, are also evaluated.

The second main part of the current volume addresses the overriding trend in changes in health and mortality: the fall in average mortality, or, in other words, the rise in average life

---

Centuries', *Historical Social Research — Quantum Information*, 15 (1980), pp. 24–39; idem, 'Zu den Veränderungen der Volksgesundheit zwischen 1870 und 1913 und ihren Determinanten in Deutschland (vor allem in Preußen)' in W. Conze and U. Engelhardt (eds). *Arbeiterexistenz im 19. Jahrhundert* (Stuttgart, 1981), pp. 235–92; idem, 'The German Petite Bourgeoisie and the Decline of Fertility: some Statistical Evidence from the Late 19th and Early 20th Centuries', *Historical Social Research — Quantum Information*, 22 (1982), pp. 15–49; idem, 'Modernisierung des Konsumverhaltens deutscher Mittel - und Unterschichten während der Zwischenkriegszeit', *Zeitschrift für Soziologie*, 14(5) (1985), pp. 400–10; idem et al. 'Ökonomischer Zwang oder schichttypischer Lebensstil? Muster der Einkommensaufbringung und - verwendung vor und nach dem Ersten Weltkrieg', in H. Thomas and F. Elstermann (eds), *Bildung und Beruf. Soziale und ökonomische Aspekte* (Berlin, 1985), pp. 159–88; idem, 'Veränderungen des Todesursachen-Panoramas und sozio-ökonomischer Wandel — Eine Fallstudie zum 'Epidemiologischen Übergang' in G. Gäfgen (ed.), *Ökonomie des Gesundheitswesens* (Schriften des Vereins für Sozialpolitik new series, vol. 159) (Berlin, 1986), pp. 73–100; A. Triebel, 'Differential Consumption in Historical Perspective', *Historical Social Research — Quantum Information*, 17 (1981), pp. 74–91; idem and C. Conrad, 'Family Budgets as Sources for Comparative Social History: Western Europe – USA 1889–1937', *Historical Social Research — Quantum Information*, 35 (1985), pp. 45–66; idem, 'Consumption Differentials and War Economy in Germany' in J. Winter and R. Wall (eds), *The Upheaval of War: Family, Work and Welfare in Europe 1914–1918* (Cambridge, 1988).

expectancy. Following the pioneering example of the group of British researchers led by Thomas McKeown[2] I am here concerned to establish to which factors of social development the decline in mortality can be attributed. During the course of the discussion it becomes clear that something approaching a satisfactory answer (although still a far from definitive one) can only be arrived at by taking into account social differences between — most importantly — the upper and middle classes, on the one hand, and the lower urban classes, on the other, and between town and country.

A different approach is adopted in Part III. Whereas, in essence, the preceding sections portray patterns of social inequality as evidence of the effects of class formation and stratification on social structures, the emphasis is now on the actions of groups, in particular of doctors. The question is to what extent and how they actively contributed to the processes described in Parts I and II in a way which might with hindsight be said to have had a long-term goal. A short concluding section attempts to review the theoretical framework in the light of the empirical findings.

Since the subject under discussion overlaps with a whole range of disciplines, I will no doubt not always be able to satisfy the relevant experts. As far as possible I shall endeavour to indicate the limits of my knowledge and insights, and otherwise refer the reader to the more detailed literature known to me. Since, however, my primary aim is to form an initial view of the various dimensions of the subject and their systematic interrelation, and to open up rather than close off discussion, I have kept footnotes to a minimum.

I would like to make it quite clear that the scope of the different sections of the study does not correspond, as it were, to their objective significance. Rather, I have expanded on points where the data at my disposal have allowed me to adopt new perspectives or led me to correct, qualify or clearly substantiate views expressed in the literature, and I have been on the whole briefer when referring to existing literature. To allow readers to follow my exposition for

---

2. See T. McKeown, *The Role of Medicine. Dream, Mirage or Nemesis?* (London, 1979); idem, *The Modern Rise of Population* (London, 1976); T. McKeown and R.G. Record, 'Reasons for the Decline of Mortality in England and Wales during the Nineteenth Century', *Population Studies*, 16 (1962-3); H.-H. Abholz also adopts this approach in 'Welche Bedeutung hat die Medizin für die Gesundheit?' in H.-U. Deppe (ed.), *Vernachlässigte Gesundheit* (Cologne, 1980); J.B. McKinlay et al, 'Mortality, Morbidity, and the Inverse Care Law' in A.L. Greer and S. Greer (eds), *Cities and Sickness, Health Care in Urban America* (Beverly Hills, 1983); an example of how McKeown's thesis is often misunderstood is given by F.W. Schwartz, 'Medizinische Versorgung versus Ernährung — Erklärungskonzepte für die historische Zunahme der Lebenserwartung. Kritische Anmerkungen zur historischen Medizinkritik von Th. McKeown', *Medizin-Mensch-Gesellschaft*, 9 (1984).

Preface

themselves or to draw more detailed conclusions, I have included a good deal of the statistical data that informed this study in the tables in the Appendix.

This book is a revision of the 1981 German edition. In particular, new publications of relevance have been added to the bibliography. I am most grateful to the many people who have helped me — directly and indirectly, and consciously and unconsciously — in producing this book, particularly my former colleagues at the Max Planck Institute for Educational Research, including Dr Uta Ottmüller and Armin Triebel, who were for a time involved in the project mentioned above. I am above all indebted to Professor Dr Wolfgang Edelstein, who for twelve years has supported my research with academic advice and unwavering human kindness. This book is dedicated to him.

Reinhard Spree
Berlin, April 1986

Introduction
A Theoretical Framework for the Impact of Class Formation and Stratification on Chances of Survival

The following is intended to set out some general theoretical premises. Not only does it define basic terms; it also indicates the relationships between the social phenomena described by them which will form the starting point for the interpretation of the statistical historical data below. This, of course, means that the results of the empirical historical investigation which are presented in this book can serve to illustrate and substantiate the conception of social inequality adopted here, and to differentiate between its constituent parts, but cannot be used to test its ultimate validity. The following social history of health in the late nineteenth and early twentieth centuries has a primarily descriptive function: it does not aim to be an original contribution to the theory of social inequality.[1]

As a first step to understanding the structures of social inequality in modern, industrial societies with market economies, they may be defined as the social distribution of all those scarce social goods which require human labour for their production, and the possession of which contributes to the stratification of human relations (i.e. principally wealth and knowledge). This definition may seem too narrow, for it focuses on the social distribution of what are termed investive goods, that is, those goods and personality traits which are used primarily to earn income or acquire wealth and which to this extent determine the individual's chances of compet-

---

1. For a representative account of the state of research, see in particular M. Haller, *Theorie der Klassenbildung und sozialen Schichtung* (Frankfurt am Main and New York, 1983); for more detail, see R. Kreckel (ed.), *Soziale Ungleichheiten* (Göttingen, 1983). The theory is applied to empirical research in M. Haller, *Klassenbildung und soziale Schichtung in Österreich. Analysen zur Sozialstruktur, sozialen Ungleichheit und Mobilität* (Frankfurt am Main and New York, 1982). H. Kaelble makes a valuable contribution to broadening this approach by adopting a socio-historical perspective in his international comparison *Industrialisation and Social Inequality in 19th Century Europe* (Leamington Spa, 1985).

ing in the economic market. 'This ignore[s] dimensions of social inequality related to the system of political rule and the use of symbolic resources, in other words to what is generally termed power structure and status differentiation.'[2] Thus structures of social inequality also include the distribution of goods and personality traits which affect the individual's opportunity to exercise power (in the broadest sense), and which are linked to the value other members of society ascribe to the individual. From this point of view, what is involved in structures of social inequality is a multi-dimensional, unequal distribution of opportunities with regard to material reproduction, the exercise of power (primarily political power), and social status.

Following on from this, it can be said, on the one hand, that such structures of social inequality are based upon the way material and immaterial resources are distributed. This is the distributive aspect of inequality. On the other hand, there is the relational aspect: certain relations always exist between the individuals and groups who are differentiated from each other as a result of distributive criteria. Within these relations, which are actively shaped by those involved, factors such as influence, esteem, and social association — or rejection and exclusion — are instrumental.

> The *distributive* aspect of social inequality provides information about the distribution not only of knowledge and wealth, but also of status and power. In this case, the latter — the two aspects typical in social relations — are not seen as 'role components' but as components of reward . . . The distributive aspect of inequality finds its expression in the particular system of institutionalised social positions which correlate with the criteria of inequality already mentioned. The *relational* aspect of social inequality, on the other hand, indicates how the members of society and social groups differentiated in this way are bound together by a system of social relations which are also institutionalised, but which are subject to continuous modification. What is involved here is the process structuring social inequality, linked both to those mechanisms which create and redefine social positions, and to those processes which channel the members of society into these positions.[3]

Two complementary processes govern the evolution of complex structures of social inequality. The first is *class formation*. It can be said to subsume those processes 'forming the framework within

---

2. J. Handl et al., *Klassenlagen und Sozialstruktur. Empirische Untersuchungen für die Bundesrepublik* (Frankfurt am Main and New York, 1977), p. 18.
3. Haller, *Theorie der Klassenbildung*, p. 32.

Introduction

which certain persons and groups attempt either individually or with the assistance of specific organisations to pursue their own interests and establish and extend positions of power in the production and distribution of socially created wealth'.[4] It is largely in commodity and labour markets that class formation takes place. The main strategies of class formation concern the creation and control of monopolies, and the influencing and shaping of power structures and the division of labour in the work place. However, there is also some overspill into the realms of government policy and the development of public opinion.

The process of class formation involves life chances that are mediated via markets.[5] Following Max Weber, it is assumed that 'the kind of chance in the *market* is the decisive moment which presents a common condition for the individual's fate.'[6] This fate, common to the lives of large groups of people, takes the form of an identical or similar position in relation to the life chances that are mediated by the market, and is defined as *class situation*. Viewed in this way, class situation is always *market situation* in relation to the resultant constellation of what are termed causal components of life chances.[7] Accordingly, class situations circumscribe people's 'differing capacities to act'.[8]

The crucial factor dividing these capacities to act is whether the actors involved own or do not own means of production. Weber speaks of propertied and acquisition classes (*Besitzklassen* and *Erwerbsklassen*), the latter characteristically not owning any means of production. This idea can be developed further by following Giddens, who recasts the term 'market situation' as *market capacity*,[9] which involves a recognition that, apart from the possession or non-possession of means of production, market-determined life chances are also considerably affected by whether or not any additional, scarce resources are at the individual's or the group's disposal. With regard to the acquisition classes, Weber did indeed note that manual and intellectual abilities or skills and formal qualifications should be included *inter alia* under scarce resources. Fundamentally, however, the sum of individual attributes can be

---

4. Ibid., p. 146.
5. See R. Dahrendorf, *Lebenschancen* (Frankfurt am Main, 1979), pp. 102-3.
6. H. Gerth and C. Wright Mills (eds), *From Max Weber. Essays in Sociology* (London, 1948), p. 182. Translation of M. Weber, *Wirtschaft und Gesellschaft. Grundriß der verstehenden Soziologie*.
7. See Weber, *Wirtschaft*, p. 181.
8. See Handl et al., *Klassenlagen*, p. 18.
9. See A. Giddens, *The Class Structure of the Advanced Societies* (London, 1973), p. 103.

counted as market capacity in so far as they can be utilised in the market process of the collective and individual exchange of — or bargaining over — life chances. This also embraces aspects of occupational status, such as the degree of autonomy and position of authority at work, which should be included since they, too, influence the individual's present and future market capacity.

More recent studies have been able to establish that, particularly when labour markets are in long-term decline, psycho-social motivations and attitudes become increasingly decisive for the market situation of those selling their labour, at least in so far as the recruitment of members of the management is concerned.[10] Even elements of life style, such as a particular mode of dress, a particular level of education, preference for certain leisure activities, or involvement in social organisations, can be components of market capacity and hence factors determining class situation.

In theory, however — that is, in times when the labour market is more or less in a state of equilibrium — psycho-social disposition and elements of life style cannot be regarded as determinants of class position: they are, rather, factors central to *stratification*. This can be understood as a process based upon esteem and the attribution of social 'honour', by which (intimate) social intercourse is restricted to individuals or groups who ascribe equal status to each other. It is thus characterised by the social evaluation of individual attributes (not only possession of goods and market chances, but also qualifications and modes of living), and by correspondingly inclusive or exclusive social action.

The process of stratification under consideration here takes place primarily in the reproductive sphere, or in 'private' life, and is, in essence, 'differential association'. This term refers to the division of the totality of social interaction into two forms. People restrict voluntary 'intimate relations' to those who are seen to be of equal status — because they share or jointly aspire to the same life styles, or hold the same values and social orientations. Unavoidable relations between people of differing status 'are limited to the level of the impersonal and neutral, and tend to be avoided'.[11] This type of stratification — differential association — makes it easier for people to achieve and secure the social status to which they aspire. It simultaneously reinforces orientations which derive from clear-cut conceptions of value, taste and relatively well-defined standards of

---

10. See P. Windolf and H.-W. Hohn, *Arbeitsmarktchancen in der Krise. Betriebliche Rekrutierung und soziale Schließung* (Frankfurt am Main and New York, 1984), pp. 114–21.
11. Haller, *Theorie der Klassenbildung*, p. 146.

behaviour, and thus allows a balanced social identity to evolve and be maintained. It may be that the individual who is continuously confronted with deviant values and goals, with a deviant life style, is confronted with a stimulating challenge. But this kind of situation is recognised as a burden which not everyone is capable of coping with — in any case not at all times — and which consequently is avoided wherever possible. It may indeed be perceived as a direct threat to one's own identity.

It appears then that stratification allows a desired social status to be acquired and maintained, and, inextricably, a social identity to be established. It is a process which does not replace class formation, but which augments it in a systematic way. It occurs primarily in the reproductive or private sphere, in other words within families and circles of friends and acquaintances, and its most important medium is life style and thus consumption, forms of socialisation and leisure interests and activities.

Having outlined the theoretical framework for my investigation, I should now like to point out the most important ways in which it relates to the subject under discussion in this book. As the expression of the ability to work, and the precondition for participation in market activities, health must be regarded as a typical resource which goes towards determining market capacity — at least for those who do not possess any means of production. In this sense, the varying degrees to which health may be impaired (illness, invalidity) can have a substantial impact on the differentiation between individuals in the acquisition classes. Of course, the social security system will compensate for some of the individual's vulnerability, but for the period we are dealing with it can be assumed that any such cushioning effect here was minimal as far as the bulk of the population was concerned. What this means is that, in accordance with the assumptions of our framework, recurring and in particular long-term illness led to differences in class situations. It can equally be expected that as a general tendency, class differences in occupational and living conditions were associated with similarly diverse health risks and degrees of vulnerability to sickness. From this it follows that an effect of class formation is to reinforce existing conditions conducive to health or ill-health. Consequently, the differences in health and mortality described below should not merely be regarded as evidence of general social inequality. Rather they indicate specifically *class* differences in the range of disposable life chances, and in the mechanisms at work in the process of class formation.

The second process structuring social inequality, as we have already noted, is stratification. Ultimately, this is linked to the Weberian category of 'status group' (*Stand*).

> In contrast to classes, status groups (*Stände*) are normally communities. They are, however, often of an amorphous kind. In contrast to the purely economically determined 'class situation' we wish to designate as 'status situation' (*ständische Lage*) every typical component of the life fate of men that is determined by a specific, positive or negative, social estimation of *honour*. This honour may be connected with any quality shared by a plurality . . .[12]

While a similar or identical class situation by no means entails necessary or regular social contact between individuals, for a status group such contact is crucial, for its members are expected to observe a particular life style. This implies that social contact is restricted on the basis of ascribed social values, and is the reason underlying our decision to define social stratification as a process of differential association.

Market capacity is by no means the sole determinant of an individual's health and susceptibility to illness, though it is also not the least important. Qualifications and occupational position and their concomitants (income, actual workloads and a specific degree of autonomy and power to issue instructions) are important factors affecting health, particularly in the case of large numbers of wage-earners. Indeed, for these people such factors are dominant. But even for manual workers — and more so for other members of the acquisition classes who are not exposed first and foremost to the harsh working conditions of manual labour — factors such as diet, clothing, housing conditions, habits and customs, and general levels of education have a considerable effect on health. This means, then, that within the social class, elements of life style go to shape patterns of health and illness. Moreover, if we bear in mind the mechanisms which operate within status groups, an individual's health or ill-health (especially certain forms of illness and invalidity) may act as criteria by which social contact is established or broken off. To this extent, social inequalities in the face of illness and death refer us back to the process of stratification, and are affected by this very process. In other words, there is continuous interaction between the elements of life style we have mentioned — which are themselves subject to social change — and inequalities in health and mortality.

12. Weber, *Wirtschaft*, p. 187.

Introduction

In order to be able to break down this matrix of interrelationships into more detail, it seems necessary, however, to analyse morbidity, the frequency of various causes of death, and mortality rates in terms of criteria which are related not only to the social structure. It would be more desirable to have additional data that would enable illness, death and the reactions of those affected, and of people in their social environment, to be interpreted as elements of life style or as criteria underlying 'differential association' (stratification). Unfortunately, however, lack of information prevents this.

A further aspect of Weber's thoughts on the concept of status groups is important for the framework adopted here. Let us take the following statement:

> For all practical purposes, stratification by status goes hand in hand with a monopolisation of ideal and material goods or opportunities, in a manner we have come to know as typical . . . As to the general *effect* of the status order . . . it is the hindrance of the free development of the market.[13]

The tendencies both to monopolise ideal and material opportunities and to limit free market development are factors which may be regarded as typical components of the professionalisation of doctors during the late nineteenth century, both in Germany and elsewhere. In addition, the attempts to determine an appropriate level of income and maintain an appropriate life style (monitored by so-called Courts of Honour) are signs that in the period under investigation doctors in Germany acted as a 'status group' in Weberian terms. Thus, a historical investigation into health not only allows us to interpret structures of social inequality as evidence of class formation and social stratification. We can also point to doctors as a group whose interests led it actively to promote processes of class formation.

As Parry and Parry have established, the professionalisation of doctors can be meaningfully analysed from the point of view of collective social mobility.[14] It is apparent that doctors' professional associations pursued policies in the interests of the status group, and that this also contributed to class formation. The medical profession was able to exclude unlicensed competitors from the market by controlling access to the profession and by autonomously

---

13. See ibid., pp. 190–3.
14. See N. Parry and J. Parry, *The Rise of the Medical Profession. A Study of Collective Social Mobility* (London, 1976), p. 56.

supervising professional practice. Other groups of healers, whose activities were defined as inferior, became dependent upon the medical profession, and the latter's market capacity gained ground at the expense of others. Status-group elements in the policy pursued by the profession also reinforced the internal homogeneity and the power of the group in the socio-political sphere. Consequently it is not only true that multiple relations exist between class differences and factors typical of status-group differentiation. It can also be said that these relations, as the example of medical professionalisation will show, can even take the form of strategies aimed at creating structures of inequality.

As was mentioned above, structures of social inequality have a third dimension — the political — which should be considered even if only in a rudimentary fashion. The outcome of class formation and stratification is increasingly influenced by, and even subordinated to, factors of social structure which are shaped by political forces. The emerging social security system and an expanding social infrastructure, which have a great impact on conditions in private reproduction, must be borne in mind. These two factors in conjunction increasingly determine the range of causal components of market capacity which individuals and groups have at their disposal. But it is not only in this way that the welfare state and infrastructural measures designed to augment and redistribute life chances intervene in and modify the processes of class formation. If allowance is made for differences between generations, it can be said that the life styles and modes of behaviour of entire social groups are recast by infrastructural features. This is particularly true where health care in the widest sense and its impact on social differences in health, morbidity and mortality are concerned. However, it can be assumed that the market capacity of certain groups also correlates with political power, particularly if a withdrawal of their services would have serious consequences for society's total reproduction.[15] To this extent it cannot be expected that welfare policies and infrastructural measures can eradicate the fundamental differences between propertied classes and acquisition classes, nor between the diverse market capacities which are assigned considerably varying values within the latter classes. It is far more likely to be the case that groups endowed with market capacities suited to

---

15. See U. Bergmann et al., 'Herrschaft, Klassenverhältnis und Schichtung' in T.W. Adorno (ed.), *Spätkapitalismus oder Industriegesellschaft? Verhandlungen des deutschen Soziologentages 1968* (Stuttgart, 1969); C. Offe, 'Tauschverhältnis und politische Steuerung. Zur Aktualität des Legitimationsproblems' in idem, *Strukturprobleme des kapitalistischen Staates* (Frankfurt am Main, 1972).

gaining political power tend to be favoured, while other wage-earning groups are relatively disadvantaged. These hypotheses must be tested against data on health and mortality, for example by examining differences between unionised and non-unionised workers.

The theoretical framework for my investigation can be briefly summarised as follows. Numerical data on health and mortality rates among the population provide a profile of structures of social inequality which simultaneously attest to processes of class formation and social stratification. Government policy involving social security measures and changes to the infrastructure can modify such structures, but it is presumed that it cannot release them entirely from their connection with market capacity. For the majority of members of what have been termed the acquisition classes (dependent wage earners), social stratification too is closely, though by no means exclusively, related to the distribution of life chances which results from different market capacities. As a result, it can be expected that class formation — i.e. the causal factors of market capacity — will have a particularly marked impact on empirically identifiable structures of social inequality. An examination of professions reveals that there are important exceptions to this, above all in the case of elite qualifications: these are scarce, highly valued by society and are thus determining factors of market capacity. In this case, class situation virtually takes on the character of a dependent variable that is largely determined by the policy pursued by an occupational status group operating in a propitious socio-economic environment.

There is no doubt that the framework outlined above goes far beyond the confines of my investigation, since it refers to the principles by which whole societies are structured. In contrast, health, sickness and mortality — the narrower focus of the present work — form only a single, albeit important dimension of the process of social reproduction. However, structured social inequality is very much in evidence in this dimension. Moreover, by examining both the factors determining health, sickness and mortality, and their social consequences, it can be quite clearly seen how the processes that structure society are enmeshed one with another. To this extent, the theoretical framework is appropriate for the subject under analysis.

There is also a sound methodological argument for elaborating the underlying conception of the structuring of social inequality in this way. Not to have done so would have meant interpreting my sources on the basis of *ad hoc* hypotheses, which would have caused

Introduction

the book to become a collection of arbitrarily structured empirical data. However, there is an enormous wealth of information, and literally millions of statistics, relating to the subject and period under discussion. It is only by reference to a theoretical framework that the statistics acquire any value for historical research, since, as it were, they are thereby transformed from items of information into *relevant data*. By consistently using our framework as a context for seemingly trivial information such as 'frequency of breast-feeding by mothers' or 'distribution of hospital beds in the administrative districts of Prussia', the corresponding statistical figures are elevated to the level of indicators of structured social inequality. To the extent that it does this, our theoretical framework not only provides a guide to the selection of empirical information, but also gives that information precisely defined socio-historical and theoretical substance.

Part I
Changes in Health and Mortality

1
Changes in the 'People's Health'

1.1 Different Approaches

This part of the book is concerned principally with changes in life expectancy in the German Empire between 1871 and 1914. During this period, the life expectancy of the average German increased markedly. Though the increase varied with age and sex (in most age groups it was greater for women than for men), it should be noted that as early as 1871–80 women in the lower age groups (i.e. up to the age of 30 or 40) could already expect to live two to three years longer than men. In both sexes, the greatest increase in life expectancy was registered among new-born babies. Their life expectancy rose by between 11 and 12 years from an expected life-span of 38.5 years in 1871–80 to 50.7 in 1910–11 for females, and from 35.6 to 47.7 for males. This amounts to more than a third of the total actual increase in life expectancy (of new-born babies) up to the present.[1] The rise in the life expectancy of 15-year-olds was approximately five years, around half that of new-born babies. For both men and women of working age, the initial figures and the respective increases were virtually the same. Among 30-year-olds, the rise was only about four years, and among 45-year-olds two to three years.

Although, as far as the increase in pure longevity is concerned, it was new-born babies and infants in particular who profited most from the fall in the mortality rates in the late nineteenth and early twentieth centuries, even the average life expectancy of the middle age groups showed a marked rise. In the light of this it is rather difficult to refute Conze's lapidary statement that 'from the middle of the century the general level of the "people's health" (*Volksgesundheit*) took an increasingly favourable turn'.[2] Other writers,

---

1. See Presse- und Informationsant der Bundesregierung (eds), *Gesellschaftliche Daten 1979*, p. 13; *Statistisches Jahrbuch für das Deutsche Reich*, vol. 38 (1919), p. 50. For a more detailed and more extensive analysis, see A.E. Imhof, *Die gewonnenen Jahre. Von der Zunahme unserer Lebensspanne seit dreihundert Jahren* (Munich, 1981).
2. W. Conze, 'Sozialgeschichte 1850–1918' in W. Zorn (ed.), *Handbuch der*

such as Ritter and Kocka, paint a similarly optimistic picture.³ However, they do also point to a number of unfavourable trends, and discuss the problems associated with a rural population surplus that other areas found difficult to absorb, the growing numbers of people working in unhealthy conditions in offices and factories, the division of towns into residential areas with different socio-economic characteristics, and, in the poorer urban areas, a fall in the standard of living combined with a growing housing shortage.

No evidence is offered, however, to underpin these statements, or to place them in any order of significance. None the less, such observations must be important to some extent because even contemporary experts of the early part of this century often referred to them. In 1913 for example, Alfons Fischer identified a number of 'unperceived consequences of social security in Germany' in his analysis of the question whether 'the physical condition of the German working population [is] still in decline'.⁴ With the help of a vast amount of statistical data, Fischer concluded that during the later years of the Empire the general level of health in the population had in fact hardly improved at all, and may even have worsened. Marxist writers, on the other hand, always answer this question in terms of a universal social theory:

> To be poor means to be sick. But to be both poor and sick is to be poor ten times over! The sick proletarian is a victim of his low standard of living, of his miserable housing conditions, of the injuries to which he is exposed at work. He has no chance of recovering unless he can escape from such terrible conditions for a long time and live in a more favourable environment. But how can he be expected to earn a higher wage or find a better place to live as long as the conditions of exploitation prevail? And how can we expect capitalism to help improve the workers' lot as long as the maximisation of profit is the goal of production? In such circumstances, being cured is out of the question. At best there is only one way out: ignore the pain, eliminate the symptoms which are causing so much trouble, and gather up enough strength to carry on living and working for the time being.⁵

---

deutschen Wirtschafts- und Sozialgeschichte (Stuttgart, 1976), vol. 2, p. 638.
  3. See G.A. Ritter and J. Kocka (eds), *Deutsche Sozialgeschichte. Dokumente und Skizzen, Band 2: 1870–1914* (Munich, 1974), p. 34.
  4. A. Fischer, 'Vermisste Folgen der deutschen Sozialversicherung. Ein Beitrag zu der Frage: Schreitet die physische Verelendung der deutschen Arbeiterbevölkerung fort?', *Jahrbücher für Nationalökonomie und Statistik*, 3rd series, vol. 46, (1913), pp. 577–602, esp. pp. 585 and 601.
  5. O. Rühle, *Illustrierte Kultur- und Sittengeschichte des Proletariats* (Berlin, 1930), vol. 1, p. 513.

In this analysis, Rühle was, on the one hand, merely reiterating one of the fundamental tenets of the Marxist labour movement, which generally does not allow itself to be influenced too much by empirical considerations. As early as 1877, the Social Democratic Party newspaper *Vorwärts* was arguing along the same lines: 'Socialism is the best, indeed the only doctor . . . by eliminating the causes of sickness, socialism will eliminate sickness.'[6] Nevertheless, Rühle did attempt to support his theses by including a wealth of statistical data on the higher mortality rate amongst workers, their greater susceptibility to illness and accidents, and the inadequacy of the medical care provided for them when they fell ill.[7] The evidence, however, remains rather fragmentary and impressionistic. In terms of time, region and age group under consideration it is extremely limited, and it is impossible to judge whether any conclusions might be universally applicable. As it stands, then, Rühle's collection of documents is not sufficient to help us establish a clearly focused picture of the 'people's health' and the changes it underwent between 1871 and 1914.

Stearns's interpretation of this whole question is different again. He assumes that, on average, the health of even the working population improved towards the end of the nineteenth century. As far as Germany is concerned, he suspects that industrial workers were basically 'better off' (except in some individual cases) than, for example, those in the technologically more backward trades — i.e. skilled manual labourers and, above all, workers in cottage industries.[8] In addition he also acknowledges the contrary evidence (which Rühle had rather too readily reduced to generalisations) provided by statistics on occupational illnesses, occupational mortality, accidents at work and the reports from workers or their representatives on significant and increasing dangers to health. None the less, he believes that it is not possible to conclude from this that the overall level of the 'people's health' had actually fallen. In his view, reports showing a deterioration in the physical condition of the working population had been misinterpreted, and he claimed instead that they were essentially a reflection of the psychi-

---

6. *Vorwärts*, 87, 27 July 1877, quoted in A. Labisch, 'Die gesundheitspolitischen Vorstellungen der deutschen Sozialdemokratie von ihrer Gründung bis zur Parteispaltung (1863–1917)', *Archiv für Sozialgeschichte*, 16 (1976), p. 341.
7. See Rühle, *Sittengeschichte*, pp. 496–523. A similar tone is adopted by Kuczynski, who, incidentally, restricts his examination to data on the frequency and causes of accidents and to occupational diseases; see J. Kuczynski, *Darstellung der Lage der Arbeiter in Deutschland von 1871 bis 1900* (Berlin, 1962), ch. 4, esp. pp. 384–7 (vol. 3 of *Die Geschichte der Lage der Arbeiter unter dem Kapitalismus*).
8. See P.N. Stearns, *Lives of Labour: Work in a Maturing Industrial Society* (London, 1975), pp. 195, 220–1, 347.

cal and mental problems faced by a working population which was coming to terms with and adapting to changing working conditions in modern industry (rationalisation, more extensive mechanisation and fragmentation of work).

Each of these different interpretations is able to call on concrete historical evidence in support. However, in each case, the empirical evidence presented is rather flimsy and is restricted above all to selective aspects of sickness and health that are not subjected to any sort of systematic analysis. For this reason, it is difficult to combine the prevailing theories, and a clear picture of the course of the 'people's health' is still lacking. Thus it would appear to be important for any further socio-historical analysis of this particular subject to make the concept of the 'people's health' easier to operate with (i.e. make it easier to measure). Above all, we need to select a suitable set of indicators that will enable us to chart the changes in health in Germany over longer periods of time. It is true that any such indicators refer to only a few aspects of social reality. However, if they are systematically organised, they can provide not only a picture of changes in health, but also a frame of reference for additional information which can be gleaned from other problematics. This is the most important way in which the following analysis differs from both contemporary studies of occupational, industrial and social hygiene, on the one hand, and the various reference books on medical statistics on the other.[9] The problems associated with selecting these kinds of indicators will be discussed in the next section.

1.2 Basic Concepts, Problems of Measurement and Sources

Health is a concept that is both universal and extremely relative. Its meaning changes not only from one historical period to another, but also within the bounds of one particular period or society, and from one subculture to another. This lack of uniformity is a consequence of the fact that health is an individual condition which is determined simultaneously by psycho-biological and socio-cultural factors. In other words, what we mean by health (or ill-health) is, on the one hand, a particular interpretation by the individual affected of various psychological and physical signals. On the other, it is a supra-individual phenomenon with a social

---

9. See particularly H. Westergaard, *Die Lehre von der Mortalität und Morbilität* (Jena, 1901), 2nd edn; F. Prinzing, *Handbuch der medizinischen Statistik* (Jena, 1906; 2nd edn, 1931).

role.[10] In modern industrial societies we tend to prefer more emphatic definitions of the concept of health. These usually revolve around a desire for well-being and happiness and for the greatest possible fulfilment of an individual's potential for personal development, all of which are felt to be entirely natural aspirations.

The early labour movement interpreted the importance of health in much more sober terms, but nevertheless identified the essence of the problem in a way that remained valid until fairly recently. The 'Basic Statutes of the German Working Men's Brotherhood' (*Grundstatuten der Deutschen Arbeiter-Verbrüderung*) of 1850 state: 'The health of the working man, the condition which above all others affects his ability to work, is, together with that ability to work, often the only, but always the most important thing he possesses.'[11] From this perspective, the concept of health is reduced to the ability to work, perceived subjectively and accepted by the standards of the social environment. Such an interpretation is perfectly justified when it is applied to the sections of the population dependent for their living on the sale of their own labour (the acquisition classes). Although the introduction and expansion of sickness insurance reduces the risk of the health of dependent wage-earners deteriorating, it does not eliminate the risk entirely. The greatest change initiated by the introduction of sickness insurance is rather the obligatory regulation of the decisions concerning which social groups are to have the right to define what 'sickness' actually is. It is well known that in the past the responsibility for this rested with doctors. In essence, they were allowed to decide who was sick and who was healthy on the basis of certain professional standards. This was certainly the case after the introduction of statutory sickness insurance, but it was even partially true before then when there were only the various (private) factory insurance and benefit funds. The consequence of this development was that public attention became increasingly focused on the ever more precisely described and more reliably diagnosed illnesses and diseases, whilst the concept of health steadily waned into an insignificant category used to classify the absence or low level of ill-health in the individual.[12]

---

10. See R. Kohn and K.L. White (eds), *Health Care. An International Study* (London, 1972), p. 2.
11. *Grundstatuten der deutschen Arbeiter-Verbrüderung, v. Februar 1850* part 3, introduction, quoted in Labisch, *Die gesundheitspolitischen Vorstellungen*, p. 332.
12. See C. v. Ferber, 'Gesellschaftliche Grundlagen der Volksgesundheit', *Arbeit und Leistung*, 25 (1971); F. Hartmann, *Wandel und Bestand in der Heilkunde I. Materialen zur Geschichte der Medizin für Studenten*, (Munich, 1977), pp. 58–62, 237–66.

Recent discussions of the indicators of health have tended to reflect this progressive tendency to minimalise the concept of health or, more properly, this failure to make it more specific and concrete. In an interesting study on the subject, Helberger has written that 'one of the primary aims of health is life itself; that is, a long life, measured in relation to average life expectancy. The second major aim is related to the "healthiness" of that life. A suitable unit of measurement would appear to be the number of days of sickness or ill-health per person per year'.[13] Viewed positively then, this seems to measure health simply in relation to the length of life. Without exception, the other indicators refer to health from a negative point of view in that they attempt to define the severity, duration and consequences of sickness. In developing a systematic pattern of these indicators, Helberger bases his work on a sliding scale of sickness ranging from objective evidence of sickness through the subjective perception of sickness, the inability to work, confinement to bed, to extended periods in hospital care and finally to death. This continuum can also be used as a point of departure for finding indicators suitable for tracing the history of the 'people's health'. Essentially, this means that we are increasingly restricted to the types of indicator that can actually be derived from source material. The next step is then to establish to what extent the initial selection has to be modified in view of the time and energy that is actually available for research.

To begin with, it seems to be worth noting that the number of objectively sick people is greater than the number of subjectively sick. This stems from the fact that the individual affected does not in every case perceive all of the objectively verifiable symptoms. However, even today the chance of recording on a statistical basis all cases of objective sickness that are not perceived subjectively are minimal. The only way is by mass screenings or routine check-ups, for example, but these occur infrequently. Up to now I have not researched this kind of statistical material, although it is available in the form of medical statistics on those entering the civil service, or from the much more specific medical examinations of conscripts which are conducted to establish their fitness for military service. At the same time, though, the number of subjectively sick people is equally difficult to establish, whether they are still fit for work or are already bed-ridden. For as long as they are not receiving medical treatment or preferably, from the point of view of the data,

---

13. C. Helberger, 'Soziale Indikatoren für das Gesundheitswesen der BRD. Ansätze, Probleme, Ergebnisse', *Allgemeines Statistisches Archiv*, 60 (1) (1976), p. 34; on the sliding scale of sickness see p. 32.

hospital care, their numbers remain unknown. It is only when medical institutions are involved — doctors and hospitals — that cases of illness are more likely to be recorded as statistics, and that this will be done in a way that allows relevant indicators to be derived.

Since our primary aim is to develop a systematic pattern of indicators with which to measure the level of health, shifts in the focus of analysis from health to sickness and the relegation of 'health' to a residual role, seem to present some problems. An additional drawback with such approaches is that sickness can also only be measured selectively. I have come to this conclusion after examining the limited possibilities of measuring sickness on the basis of current statistical records and methods. It is fair to say that the actual chances of establishing a set of indicators for the late nineteenth and early twentieth centuries are even slimmer.

> Although studies of ill-health generally should include the total population, data are only ever recorded on individual illnesses or groups of illnesses. More comprehensive statistical analyses of sickness only exist for certain sections of the population. The major sources in this respect are reports of officially notifiable diseases, statistical surveys compiled by the various social insurance institutions and the different public service organisations such as the Army, Navy, Police and Post Office, and, finally, statistical reports of child-absenteeism from school.[14]

If we leave aside the public service organisations, because they represented no more than a negligible proportion of the total population, and statistics on school absenteeism, because these did not begin to be compiled in a reliable way until after the First World War, then the only sources remaining are statistics on sickness insurance and reports of notifiable diseases. The latter refer to an extremely small number of mainly infectious diseases — epidemics — that were felt to be particularly dangerous. However, as we shall show later, by the second half of the nineteenth century, these had already become surprisingly insignificant, at least in the context of the total number of deaths registered.

For their part, the value of sickness insurance statistics is impaired by the fact that they failed to register the cases of ill-health that did not render the sufferer unfit for work. Nor did they distinguish between those who were suffering from relapses and

---

14. W. Gajewski, 'Statistik der Krankheiten und Gebrechen einschließlich der Krankenanstaltsstatistik' in F. Burgdörfer (ed.), *Die Statistik in Deutschland nach ihrem heutigen Stand. Ehrengabe für Friedrich Zahn* (Berlin, 1940), vol. 1, p. 302.

those who were ill for the first time, with the result that some cases may have been counted twice. Finally, one particular drawback is that it is impossible to establish whether those cases who were no longer paid sickness insurance (i.e. after the statutory benefit period had expired) had died from the illness recorded in the statistics, or how long the illness had lasted.[15] Thus any attempts to interpret available data on sickness insurance will have to take into account the considerable gaps and uncertainties inherent within them, all of which is hardly likely to make the effort involved in processing the data seem worthwhile.

Another kind of approach to establishing indicators for charting the development of the 'people's health' stems from contemporary interpretations of the late nineteenth and early twentieth centuries:

> We live in an age of medical discoveries, progress in public health and hygiene standards, and movements for social reform. This then prompts the question of whether the general level of health has actually improved, and if so, whether this improvement can be measured statistically. One yardstick — in fact, the only reliable yardstick given the present state of statistical analysis — for measuring the level of public health is the population's average mortality rate.[16]

Written in 1897, this statement coincided exactly with the tide of specialist opinion that had prevailed since the 1860s. In 1877, for instance, the Imperial Health Office (*Kaiserliches Gesundheitsamt*), founded the previous year, began producing its weekly publication (*Veröffentlichungen des Kaiserlichen Gesundheitsamtes*). One of the most important regular features was entitled 'Bulletin on the state of health and the course of epidemic diseases (*Volkskrankheiten*)'.[17] This column continued to appear right up until the First World War. Various infectious diseases were referred to as 'epidemic diseases' (*Volkskrankheiten*), but the reports generally concentrated

---

15. See Gajewski, 'Statistik', p. 306; Prinzing, *Handbuch*, 2nd edn, pp. 193–4, 200–9, 223–36. Equally difficult to use are the following large-scale regional surveys: *Frankfurter Krankheitstafeln*, no. 4 in new series of *Beiträge zur Statistik der Stadt Frankfurt am Main* (Frankfurt am Main, 1900); Kaiserliches Statistisches Amt (eds), *Krankheits- und Sterblichkeitsverhältnisse in der Ortskrankenkasse für Leipzig und Umgebung. Untersuchungen über den Einfluß von Geschlecht, Alter und Beruf*, 4 vols (Berlin, 1910). Both works are based on data for comparatively long periods, but only averages for the periods were published. Much could be gained from analysing archive material on sickness insurance funds, but this would have to be a separate piece of research limited to specific regions.
16. W. Kruse, 'Die Verminderung der Sterblichkeit in den letzten Jahrzehnten und ihr jetziger Stand', *Zeitschrift für Hygiene und Infectionskrankheiten*, 25 (1897), p. 113.
17. *Veröffentlichungen des Kaiserlichen Gesundheitsamtes* (1877 onwards), vol. 1 onwards, p. 1.

on the number of deaths that resulted from these illnesses rather than the total number of cases. The weekly statistical summaries of the causes of death regularly contained information on the numbers of people who had died from measles, German measles, scarlet fever, diphtheria and croup, typhoid, child-bed fever, tuberculosis (*Lungenschwindsucht*), acute infections of the respiratory organs, and diarrhoea with vomiting (*Brechdurchfall*). The number of deaths caused by smallpox, cholera, typhus, relapsing fever, epidemic cerebrospinal meningitis, rabies, whooping cough and erysipelas (*Rose*) was published as one figure because even as early as the late 1870s they were the cause of no more than a few fatalities. In view of our efforts to establish parameters which can profitably be used as instruments for direct observation and measurement, it seems particularly significant that the overall level of health in the population was felt to be accurately reflected by the relative mortality rates associated with the 'epidemic diseases' — that is, the relative frequency of certain causes of death and the way they developed over a certain period of time.

It is clear, then, that contemporary observers equated health purely and simply with being alive — or at least with survival. The fact that greater efforts were made to register the number of deaths and, in particular, what caused them, rather than to record morbidity or the frequency of particular diseases, was probably prompted by the high average mortality rate. We have to bear in mind the combined effect of the massive threat of death which hung over many people, on the one hand, and the impotence of doctors in the face of the majority of illnesses (and the infectious diseases in particular), on the other. Infectious or epidemic diseases moved to the forefront of medical attention in the second half of the nineteenth century, assuming the legacy left by the great epidemics of the pre-industrial era which, for reasons that have yet to receive adequate scientific explanation, became so rare after 1800. It is therefore quite understandable that the public health officials in the Imperial Health Office regarded 'health' as the ability to live a prolonged life, or, in other words, as the relative absence of 'epidemic' diseases. In view of the lack of effective medical treatment, it was easy to measure the incidence of these diseases reliably by counting the deaths caused by them.

However, between 1870 and 1914, the situation changed with the result that such emphasis on infectious diseases no longer seemed to be justified. This cannot have escaped the attention of the medical statisticians of the day. The changes were threefold. Firstly, doctors were increasingly in a position to provide effective treatment. Secondly, various infectious diseases became less and less important, for a number of reasons that will be outlined below. In other words, other causes of death began to deserve more attention. Thirdly, the overall mortality rate fell by so much that it became increasingly less plausible to conclude that the frequency of a particular cause of death was an accurate reflection of the overall number of people suffering from the corresponding illness. None the less, until the end of the 1930s, the experts remained convinced that the statistics recording causes of death were an important indicator of morbidity, as the following quotation shows:

> In the German Empire, as in every other civilised country no doubt, statistics on causes of death represent the most important health statistic . . . [Despite a shift of interest in the medical profession], those wishing to study particular illnesses, or to evaluate the health of certain sections of the population, continue to base their analyses primarily on these figures. It is impossible to make a conclusive assessment of the level of popular health without recourse to the statistics on the causes of death. For the time being, there is no other single type of statistical health survey that comes near to achieving anything like the same comprehensiveness and numerical stability.[18]

This view is based above all on their 'comprehensiveness' and 'numerical stability'. In this respect, the quality of the statistics on causes of death really did improve considerably in the first decades of the twentieth century. In the decades before that they had been just about adequate but by no means satisfactory, as we shall see below. Nevertheless, for the period that concerns us, the mortality statistics, including the causes of death, represented by far the most sophisticated and reliable information on popular health available at that time — and were at any rate far superior to the rather crude statistics on morbidity.

Following the contemporary view, I shall now proceed to examine the changes that took place in the 'people's health' during the late nineteenth and early twentieth centuries by examining statistical data on mortality. I shall begin with the average mortality rate for the whole of the German Empire, which, as I shall show, is in need of considerable refinement. Age, region, size of community and causes of death are appropriate criteria by which to break the figures down systematically. Our intention is to combine and observe these criteria over the longest possible period. Conse-

18. E. Meier, 'Statistik der Todesursachen' in Burgdörfer, *Statistik in Deutschland*, p. 289.

quently, the fact that no statistical surveys of the causes of death were conducted at national level before 1892 means that we are obliged to concentrate on the regional data that is available. In this respect, Prussia seems to be the ideal object for a comparison over time, and one which avoids the problems associated with redefining the various analytical categories and with the different survey techniques. It also enables us to study rural areas as well as cities and towns. It was by far the largest German state with highly developed statistical records of the causes of death. More importantly, perhaps, the analytical categories and survey procedures remained constant between 1875 and 1902. The changes in the nomenclature used to describe the causes of death that were introduced in 1902–3 make it more difficult, though not impossible, to continue the chronological comparison as far as 1913. At the same time, though, there is little sense in extending the comparison back to the period before 1875 because the nomenclature used between 1816 and 1874 was completely different to the new (and modernised) terminology used later on. There is one important drawback with the Prussian statistics that ought, however, to be mentioned: in most cases a post-mortem examination was not required by law, which implies that a high percentage of the causes of death were presumably established without a doctor being present. To what extent this might have reduced the value of the statistics has not yet been calculated conclusively.

As I demonstrated above, my indicators have not been chosen by combining a large number of different types of data into a single, constructed relationship. Instead, I select one basic indicator — mortality rate — which is then analysed systematically by breaking the figures down according to a number of different criteria. Even if the analysis is restricted to a small number of differential criteria (age, region, size of community, cause of death), the calculations involved quickly reach such proportions that they simply cannot be carried out in a reasonable length of time. As a rule, one calculation generally leads directly to the next because each new level of information immediately prompts a large number of new questions. The basic statistics (the annual number of deaths classified according to 15 different age groups, 36 administrative districts, a large number of towns and rural districts and 30 causes of death) was published regularly in the series *Preußische Statistik*. However, they were rarely subjected to any sort of systematic analysis. I have thus been obliged to restrict my initial evaluations to a few sample years, administrative districts or towns, together with a small selection of significant causes of death. The two main years selected for comparison are

1876 and 1901 (years when the state of the 'people's health' was normal, and yet which provide a solid statistical basis because they immediately followed years in which a census had been carried out). The comparison is continued, in part at least, up to 1913, with the year 1903 inserted as a transitional year, since it was then that the new nomenclature for the causes of death was introduced.

The Prussian averages are compared with those of the administrative districts of Königsberg and Gumbinnen, on the one hand, and Arnsberg and Düsseldorf, on the other. I also include four major cities in my analysis: Berlin, Dortmund, Essen and Frankfurt am Main. For certain questions a summary has been made of the figures available for the 22 Prussian cities which by 1900 had more than 100,000 inhabitants. In analysing these differences between the various regions and sizes of community, I have tried to classify the mortality statistics in such a way that it becomes possible to assess to what extent the figures concern the lower social strata and working classes. The reason for this is connected with the fact that 'people's health' refers essentially to these especially large social groups about which there is a relative lack of readily available representative information. Unfortunately, the mortality statistics do not contain any information that may be linked directly to features of social stratification. (An exception to this are the statistics available for infant mortality which will be discussed in greater detail below.) This failing can only be compensated for by adopting a method of data analysis which will enable us to touch on social groups indirectly. In order to draw plausible conclusions about particular social groups, it may be helpful to select certain age groups and examine the incidence among them of particular causes of death.

Since I am interested in deducing to what extent the working classes were (directly) affected, objections could be raised to the fact that I am preoccupied with the concept of the 'people's health' and general mortality rates and have failed to delve into the enormous quantities of statistics available on industrial and occupational health. However, the very quantity of this kind of literature obscures the fact that genuinely useful statistical data containing reliable information on both the relative dangers to health associated with certain occupations and their mortality rates (classified according to causes of death), are in fact extremely scarce. It is almost invariably presented as a jumble of data showing the number of cases of sickness or death in certain occupations, occasionally classified according to types of illness or cause of death, but without reference to the total number of cases. Prinzing, the famous medical statistician, was moved by this situation to conclude: 'There is no other activity in the field of public health that has produced so much useless statistical material as studies of occupational health.'[19] Moreover, the figures that are published lack uniformity with respect to both region and time, with the result that, by and large, it is impossible to arrive at a systematic description of health or sickness in the various occupational groups, let alone any sort of chronological pattern. Thus, although it would seem to be extremely sensible in theory to exploit this particular type of source, an examination of a representative selection of material shows it would be somewhat unprofitable in practice.

1.3 Changes in Mortality Rates and the Course of the 'People's Health'

From the comments above on changes in life expectancy, it can be said that the average mortality rate in Imperial Germany must have fallen markedly in the course of the period under discussion. Ignoring the 'surges' in 1866 and 1871 caused by the Austro-Prussian and Franco-Prussian Wars, the average mortality rate reached its highest point in the nineteenth century at the beginning of the 1870s (in 1872–3 there were on average 28.7 deaths per 1000 people) and then fell rapidly. By 1913 it had fallen by almost half (15 per 1000).[20] The most important component of the average rate in the nineteenth century was the level of infant mortality, which regularly lay between 25 and 35 per cent. In view of this high percentage, and if we recall that the average life expectancy of new-born babies had increased considerably by 1913, it is clear that the level of infant mortality must also have fallen. It is worth noting, however, that it was not until the turn of the century that it

---

19. F. Prinzing, 'Die Gesundheitsstatistik', in R. Abel (ed.), *Handbuch der praktischen Hygiene* (Jena, 1913), vol. 1, p. 31; see idem, *Handbuch*, 1st edn, pp. 473ff. For individual results see idem, *Handbuch*, 2nd edn, pp. 254–64, and cited works. Even in a recent attempt at a social history of occupational illnesses and medicine, which is otherwise a piece of work which should be applauded, there are many shortcomings in the analysis of statistical data: see R. Müller and D. Milles (eds), *Beiträge zur Geschichte der Arbeiterkrankheiten und der Arbeitsmedizin in Deutschland* (Schriftenreihe der Bundesanstalt für Arbeitsschutz, Sonderschrift 15), (Dortmund, 1984); idem, Berufsarbeit und Krankheit (Frankfurt am Main and New York, 1985); P Weindling (ed.), *The Social History of Occupational Health* (London, 1985).
20. See W.G. Hoffman et al., *Das Wachstum der deutschen Wirtschaft seit der Mitte des 19. Jahrhunderts* (Berlin, 1965), pp. 172ff. For a promising theory for interpreting such data see also A. Omran, 'Epidemiologic Transition in the US. The Health Factor in Population Change', *Population Bulletin*, 32 (2) (1977); idem, 'The Epidemiologic Transition. A Theory of Epidemiology of Population Change', *Milbank Memorial Fund Quarterly*, 49 (1) (1971), pp. 509–38.

began to fall at the same rate as the overall average mortality rate. The national infant mortality rate stagnated at between 20 and 23 per cent in the period before 1885, and by 1900 had declined by no more than 2 percentage points. It was not until after the turn of the century (often dated from 1906 onwards) that the level of infant mortality began to fall significantly. By the outbreak of war in 1914 it had fallen by 7 or 8 percentage points as compared with the 1870s. These figures show that initially the factors affecting the average mortality rate were felt most among adults, then, after no more than a short delay, among children and teenagers. After a lag of 20–30 years they began to have an impact on infants. Even so, by 1913 the reduction in the infant mortality rate had become so great that it clearly affected the increase in life expectancy much more than other factors that reduced the average mortality rate in all of the higher age groups between 1900 and 1913. An important contributory factor may well have been the decline in the birth-rate, which for the years preceding 1900 can still be interpreted, with some justification, as part of a cyclical phenomenon but which began to exhibit a general downward trend after the turn of the century. The fall in the birth-rate reduced the percentage of those age groups in the population that are particularly susceptible to sickness (infants and young children). Thus, after 1900, the factors that directly affected the health of infants and young children (in this context, see Chapter 2) combined with the drop in the birth-rate to bring about the sharp fall in the average mortality rate.

Figures can also be used to demonstrate how important the time-lag was before the level of infant mortality began to fall sharply. In 1876 the average mortality rate in Prussia was 27.5 per 1000 for men and 23.8 for women. However, if the figures for infants under the age of 12 months are excluded, the average mortality rate then comes to no more than 18.7 for men and 16.9 for women.[21] Although the level of infant mortality was slow to fall, it then dropped very rapidly, and by a disproportionately high amount for our period. This is reflected in the following figures: in 1913 the average mortality rates in Prussia were 15.7 in males and 14.3 in females. Without the figures for infant mortality, these figures were no more than 11.0 for males and 10.7 for females. A comparison with the 1876 levels shows that the overall mortality

21. From *Preußische Statistik*, vol. 46 (Berlin, 1878), p. xviii. For 1913 from *Medizinal-statistische Mitteilungen aus dem Kaiserlichen Gesundheitsamte*, vol. 19 (Berlin, 1917), p. 48. Standard figures on mortality rates are given, with distortions arising from the age structure of the population compensated for. For men the divergence from the original mortality rate is 0 per cent, for women 1 per cent. Cf. ibid., pp. 42–3.

rate in males had declined by 11.8 per cent but only by 7.7 per cent if infant mortality rates are excluded. The overall rate for women fell by 9.5 per cent or, omitting infant mortality, 6.2 per cent. If one wished to infer from these figures that a change in the overall level of health had taken place, one would have to conclude that, in view of the fall in the average mortality rate, it had improved gradually but tangibly since the 1870s. On the other hand, the health of infants, and the living conditions of the vast majority of the population that affected it, did not really change for the better until after the turn of the century.

The various patterns of change in the health of different age groups can be illustrated more clearly. Table 1 (to be found, with all the other tables, in the Appendix) shows the mortality rates calculated for three sample years (1876, 1901 and 1913), and classified according to five age groups and eight different regions (four administrative districts and four cities). Three significant features of changes in the mortality rate are immediately clear: the overriding significance of infant mortality; the relatively low mortality rates in young and middle-age groups compared to infants and old people; and the considerable degree of regional variation in the mortality rates in all age groups. The implications of all this become clearer if we concentrate on the rates of change in the mortality rates of different age groups in the four selected Prussian administrative districts between 1876 and 1913.[22] The table shows that in this period the fall in the mortality rate was greatest among those aged between one and 15 years. In the Prussian state as a whole, as well as in the individual administrative districts, it fell by at least two-thirds — and in the administrative district of Düsseldorf by as much as 71 per cent.

If we divide up the period under discussion into two parts (1876–1901 and 1901–13), two trends in the mortality rates stand out: the level of infant mortality did not fall to any significant degree until after 1901; and, in all other age groups, by contrast, the fall that was recorded between 1876 and 1913 mainly occurred during the last decades of the nineteenth century.

For the 1–15 age group, the districts of Königsberg and Gumbinnen were exceptions here: in these areas, the level of mortality fell at a faster rate after 1901 than it had done before the turn of the century. The district of Gumbinnen also proved to be an exception in the 15–30 age group. Since Gumbinnen was the most traditionally

---

22. See the rates of change and excess mortality rates in table form in Spree, 'Volksgesundheit', Tables 4 and 5.

agrarian area of the four, it would be reasonable to conclude that its economic and social backwardness can be held responsible for weakening the effects of the factors which contributed towards the sharp fall in the mortality rates in the other Prussian districts after 1875.

By 1913 the average mortality rate had fallen by approximately one-third in the Eastern districts and almost half in the West. After the 1–15 age group, it was adults of working age (15–60) who underwent the most dramatic change. Again, the administrative district of Düsseldorf stands out because it boasts the sharpest fall in the mortality rates of the middle age groups. Between 1876 and 1913 the drop in the mortality rate in Arnsberg, and thus any associated improvement in general levels of health, began to lag behind developments in other regions and in Prussia as a whole — most markedly in the 1–15 and 15–30 age groups, but least of all in the 30–60 age group. Perhaps this was a reflection of a widely recognised consequence of migration: internal migration benefited the highly industrialised areas by bringing to them large numbers of people who were not only from the middle age groups, but also presumably in particularly good health. At the same time, though, it should also be noted that in 1870 the mortality rate in all age groups (except infants) in Arnsberg was also the highest. In this sense, then, nothing changed before 1913.

The comparatively unfavourable health situation in Arnsberg cannot simply be blamed on the relatively high percentage of working-class inhabitants. In fact, this argument can be discounted in view of the fact that Düsseldorf, an area with a similarly high level of industrialisation, was the healthiest. The differences in the respective mortality rates therefore do not correlate either with differences in the levels of industrialisation, types of trade involved or relative size of the wage-earning population.

From an examination of the way the mortality rates vary according to the age group and region involved, it may be concluded that the extent to which changes in mortality rates in specific age groups affected the overall fall in the average between 1876 and 1913 varied considerably. A number of regional differences were superimposed on these variations. These were most marked in infant mortality and in the average rates for all age groups. The more heavily industrialised administrative districts in the West enjoyed a mortality rate that was lower than the Prussian average, whilst the relatively unfavourable situation in the Eastern provinces steadily worsened.

A plausible explanation for this discrepancy between the Eastern and Western administrative districts of Prussia might well be traced back not merely to the contrast between industry and agriculture, but also to that between town and country. The Western districts had a far greater concentration of towns, and Arnsberg in particular was remarkable even by comparison with Düsseldorf for its high level of urban agglomeration. Our hypothesis is that in the late nineteenth century the overall level of health in the towns gradually began to make up the ground it had lost in this respect to the rural areas. Table 2 shows the results of an attempt to test the plausibility of this hypothesis. Mortality rates in different age groups (in this case 15 different age groups) for 22 Prussian cities between 1876 and 1900 have been compared with those of the Prussian state as a whole. The most important results are as follows:

(1) In 1876 urban mortality rates, whether this applied to individual age groups or the average for the total urban population, were much higher than the Prussian average. Exceptions to this were figures for the 10- to 15-year-olds and 20- to 25-year-olds which, in the cities, remained slightly below the Prussian average.

(2) By 1900 a number of important changes had taken place, which only rarely attracted attention in the literature on the subject. By that time, the cities had begun to benefit from an average mortality rate that was lower (even after excluding the infant mortality figure) than the Prussian average. However, this should not lead us to conclude that health in the cities had improved by so much that the urban mortality rates were now always lower than those in the rural areas. A closer examination of the individual age groups listed in Table 2 will show that in certain age groups, mortality rates were higher in the cities. Exceptions to this were the 10- to 30-year-olds, few of whom died in the cities. Even so, by comparison with 1876, there were more urban age groups with a lower mortality rate.

(3) As far as chances of survival were concerned, the advantages enjoyed by young urban adults of working age continued.[23] However, until the mid-1920s, 30 continued to be the age beyond which the mortality rate was higher in the cities. On the other hand, in the ensuing years even the under-tens (including infants) in the cities were fortunate enough to have a mortality rate that was lower than both the Prussian average and the figures for agrarian areas.

These developments prompt the conclusion that life in the cities was affected by a number of different factors which had an ambiva-

---

23. See Prinzing, *Handbuch*, 2nd edn, p. 569, for examples for the periods 1909–12 and 1924–6.

lent effect on the health and the mortality rates of their inhabitants. From the beginning of the twentieth century onwards, those in the youngest age groups were more likely to survive, and by the First World War this was also true for young working adults. All of this seems to suggest that health improved overall. The fall in the mortality figures among all age groups, even in urban areas, suggests that these factors, in conjunction with more general influences which increased life expectancy in both town and country, also affected mortality among older working people. However, mortality among town-dwellers over 30 continued to fall more slowly than in Prussia as a whole and, presumably, than in the predominantly agricultural regions in particular. It is likely that an urban and industrial environment impaired health much more, and thus tended to raise the mortality rate. However, such environmental influences on health and mortality were not such that they directly led to sickness or death at an early age: mortality rates amoung the under-30s do not bear this out. Instead, their effect appears to have been cumulative and was 'amplified' over an extended period of time because in the cities the mortality rate grew from being almost 9 per cent higher than the Prussian average for the 30–40 age group to 16 per cent higher for the 50–60 age group, and then only to fall again for the over-60s. In the following section I shall not be able to provide an adequate explanation of the ambivalent nature of these factors, but I hope nevertheless that I shall manage to cast more light on the matter by extending our analysis to the changing pattern of the causes of death.

1.4 Changes in the Pattern of Causes of Death

Infectious diseases are generally considered to have been the most widespread cause of death in nineteenth-century Germany. This view has been held for over 100 years and has been reinforced by whole generations of physicians, medical statisticians and historians. For reasons outlined above, infectious diseases remained the primary object of attention for the medical profession from the point of its emergence right up to the First World War. There was scarcely a single medical history published at the time in which the 'fight against infectious diseases' was not romanticised and placed in the limelight, and hardly any statistical surveys that did not emphasise the importance of infectious diseases to such an extent that it is now difficult to establish the statistical patterns of any other illnesses or causes of death.

An instructive example of this is the volume entitled *Das Deutsche Reich in gesundheitlicher und demographischer Beziehung* which was published jointly by the Imperial Health Office and the Statistical Office in 1907. The most important contribution was a summary of the 'Population trends in German towns with 15,000 or more inhabitants' which contained a breakdown of all deaths between 1877 and 1904, classified according to a total of 13 different causes, nine of which were chronic and acute infectious diseases.[24] Of the remainder, three fell into the category of 'violent death' (accidents, suicides and murder), leaving a disproportionately large number of different causes of death under the single, rather uninformative (13th) heading 'All other diseases'. In 1877 this collective category accounted for almost 54 per cent of all deaths and by 1904 this had risen to almost 56 per cent. If the 2.7 per cent that referred to violent deaths are substracted from the 1877 figures, then it can be said that nine known fatal diseases accounted for 44 per cent of all deaths. In fact, 34 per cent were caused by three alone: tuberculosis (approximately 14 per cent), acute infections of the respiratory organs (11 per cent) and acute intestinal disorders (9 per cent). In 1877, measles, German measles, diphtheria, croup, scarlet fever, typhus and child-bed fever accounted for less than 10 per cent of all deaths (at least in the sections of the population covered specifically by the statistics). However, these acute infectious diseases, together with tuberculosis, generated the most interest in medical research, health policy and public health. By 1904 the percentage of all deaths caused by these diseases had fallen to under 5 per cent (this was the date when the statistics became considerably more representative). Conversely, the percentage of deaths that had been caused by pulmonary TB, acute infections of the respiratory organs and chronic intestinal disorders had risen to almost 37 per cent. Whereas other infectious diseases appear to have been statistically negligible, these belonged to the category of 'great killers' which will be examined in greater detail below. Moreover, this initial survey of statistics on causes of death during the period under discussion makes it clear that, where possible, it will be necessary to draw on material that is rather more sophisticated. It is obviously unsatisfactory if the causes of the majority of deaths are either unspecified or unknown.

In order to systematise research on the 'great killers', I have

---

24. *Das deutsche Reich in gesundheitlicher und demographischer Beziehung*, dedicated to the participants of the XIVth International Congress on Hygiene and Demography, Berlin 1907, by the Kaiserliches Gesundheitsamt and the Kaiserliches Statistisches Amt (Berlin, 1907), pp. 42–3.

compiled data on all of the illnesses and diseases which, in the years 1876, 1901 and 1913, accounted for at least 3 per cent of male deaths in Prussia.[25] In 1876, a total of rather more than 75 per cent of all male deaths in Prussia were caused by the eight diseases named above and the collective category of unspecified or unknown afflictions. Of these, the first group account for 62.1 per cent. Three of these causes of death — convulsions, congenital weakness (*angeborene Lebensschwäche*) and atrophy — almost exclusively affected infants in their first year. Infirmity, on the other hand, is associated with the over-60s. This leaves four causes of death that may be described as the 'great killers' of those between the ages of one and 60, namely tuberculosis, pleurisy or pneumonia (*Lungen-/Brustfellentzündung*), diphtheria or croup (*Diphtherie/Krupp*) and strokes (*Schlagfluß*). In 1876 these accounted for approximately 27 per cent of all deaths, with tuberculosis and pneumonia or pleurisy by far the most common of these. Like the great epidemics of old (smallpox, cholera, yellow fever, dysentery, etc.), the remaining infectious diseases, at least as far as all age groups of the male population were concerned, did not play any significant role as 'killers' after the mid-1870s.

In 1901, however, 70 per cent of all deaths were caused by nine illnesses. Compared to 1876 there were only slight changes in the composition of the 'great killers'. Atrophy and diphtheria, including croup, fell below the 3 per cent mark, whilst diarrhoea with

25. See Spree, 'Volksgesundheit', Tables 7.1 and 7.2 for information on the 'great killers'. The comparatively low relevance criterion of 3 per cent was necessary in order to take into account causes of death among the middle age groups, and not only the causes of death among infants and young children and old people, which accounted for a large proportion of all deaths. Definitions of causes of death in the text and in the tables are as follows. Up to 1903 'tuberculosis' also includes 'miliary tuberculosis' and 'tuberculosis of other organs'. However, from the statistical data for the Reich, which lists these diseases separately after 1892, it can be gathered that they usually accounted for less than 10 per cent of all deaths from 'tuberculosis of the lung'. For 1913 tuberculosis means only TB of the lung. Often 'convulsions' are included under gastric and intestinal diseases, for they are supposed to result from them. Medical historians doubt whether this is entirely certain. 'Convulsions' could also have developed from feverous diseases of another kind. At the moment there is insufficient evidence to be able to distribute the figures for deaths caused by 'convulsions' among other categories with any degree of certainty. I am grateful to Johanna Bleker for pointing this out. Up to 1903 the column 'Gastric and intestinal diseases' includes 'Atrophy' and 'Diarrhoea in children' and 'Indigenous vomiting and diarrhoea'; for 1913 'Gastric and intestinal catarrh', 'Vomiting and diarrhoea' and 'Other diseases of the digestive organs'. 'Other diseases of the respiratory organs' includes 'Inflammation of the trachea and lung catarrh', 'Pneumomnia and pleurisy' and 'Other pulmonary diseases' up to 1903; for 1913 it includes 'Pneumonia' and 'Diseases of the respiratory organs'. Up to 1903 'Cardiac and circulatory diseases' includes 'Articular rheumatism' (on this cf. *Preußische Statistik*, vol. 43 (Berlin, 1877), p. xv; Kruse, 'Verminderung', p. 123), 'Dropsy' and 'Cardiac diseases'; for 1913 'Diseases of the circulatory organs'.

vomiting in children rose above it. If we subtract from these calculations the causes of death that are usually associated with infants or the elderly (convulsions, congenital weakness, diarrhoea with vomiting and infirmity), together with the group of undetermined causes of death, all that remain are three identifiable 'great killers' of people between the ages of one and 60 which accounted for 22.4 per cent of all deaths: tuberculosis, pleurisy or pneumonia, and strokes. The threat posed by tuberculosis had receded since 1876 but deaths from acute infections of the respiratory organs had increased. The percentage of those who died from strokes remained unchanged. A further noticeable 'structural constant' was the fact that in 1901 the major causes of infant mortality that attacked the gastro-intestinal tract (convulsions, atrophy, diarrhoea with vomiting) were responsible for the same proportion of mortalities as in 1876 — a little over 24 per cent of male deaths. A breakdown by age group of the number of deaths caused by each illness will demonstrate how significant this phenomenon was for the persistently high level of infant mortality which remained unchanged until the beginning of the twentieth century.

By 1913, around 86 per cent of all deaths were caused by 13 different illnesses, each accounting for at least 3 per cent of the total. The impression is that the number of major causes of death had risen. To put this into perspective, however, it must be emphasised that a new nomenclature to describe the causes of death had been introduced after 1901. It differed from the previous one to the extent that the rather broad categories used hitherto (such as tuberculosis, infections of the respiratory organs, digestive and nervous disorders) were now further broken down. Moreover, in the intervening period diagnostic techniques had become more reliable, with the result that the significance of the 'great killers' could now only be roughly estimated by collating the data for causes of death which were now being listed separately. This was particularly true of the most important causes of infant mortality, which, like convulsions, for example, were no longer classified as a cause of death.

If we attempt to make some sense of this information, the first thing to come to our attention is that the 'great killers' mentioned above were still causing many deaths in all age groups between one and 60. Pulmonary tuberculosis (although it was no longer classified with other types of tuberculosis), together with pneumonia (again more specific than the category of pneumonia or pleurisy) accounted for an overall average of 16.5 per cent of deaths in all age groups in 1913 (in 1876 it had caused 16.4 per cent and in 1901 17.6

per cent). Overall, the proportion of deaths caused by diseases of the respiratory organs had increased by 1913 (to 22 per cent). The percentage of deaths caused by infirmity remained unchanged, while the figures for infections or illnesses of the digestive organs had fallen. However, since the latter were still responsible for 11.6 per cent of all deaths, they were still significant. It is particularly interesting to look at the category of 'great killers' that began to emerge, or at least dramatically to increase in importance in the early 1900s. These were cardiac and circulatory diseases, cancer and various nervous disorders. We should thus note that changes were taking place in the range of causes of death at the beginning of the twentieth century, even though a number of important 'structural constants' remained. This will become clearer once we have classified these findings according to age group.

The first group I have selected for more detailed evaluation is the group of 30- to 60-year-old adults. In view of the fact that during the period under discussion health meant largely the ability to work, which, in turn, was decisive in determining the individual's market capacity, these people seem especially interesting. Any diseases that accounted for at least 3 per cent of deaths in this age group in the sample years 1876 and 1913 were included in surveys. For 1876, the analysis is helped because no additional calculations have to be made in order to divide up this age group into three sections. For 1913, though, it is only possible to calculate the averages for the whole age group. At the beginning of this period, in 1876, the most common cause of death among 30- to 40-year-olds was tuberculosis, accounting for 39.4 per cent. This was followed by pleurisy and pneumonia, together with the other pulmonary diseases which, taken together, caused 10.3 per cent of the deaths in this group. This meant that in 1876 around 50 per cent of all deaths in this age group were caused by diseases of the respiratory tract. Among 40- to 50- and 50- to 60-year-olds the combined percentages for these diseases were only slightly lower (46.1 and 42 respectively). Whereas death from tuberculosis in these higher age groups became slightly less common, the number of deaths caused by the other diseases of the respiratory organs was higher. Similarly, the importance of strokes (9.5 per cent) and dropsy (*Wassersucht*) (a rather ill-defined cause of death, which rose to 6 per cent in the highest age groups) increased with age.

On top of all these there was one further cause of death deserving mention, but which has been all but ignored in this study so far. A breakdown by age group of all causes of death shows that among the 30- to 40-year-olds 7.5 per cent of all male deaths in 1876 were the result of accidents. Accidents were responsible for slightly fewer deaths in the higher age groups, but for even more among the younger groups. In the 10–15 age group they accounted for 9.3 per cent, and in the 15–20 age group as much as 12.4 per cent. Presumably, it is correct to assume that this high mortality rate from accidents was a consequence of the relatively large numbers of boys and young men being employed in trades and industries with low safety records. It is possible that as they grew older male workers tended to avoid such occupations as far as possible or, alternatively, that their greater experience helped more of them to avoid becoming involved in fatal accidents. All in all, in the three sections of the age group under discussion (30–60), a maximum of eight named causes were responsible for at least 70 per cent of all deaths throughout the period. With the exception of typhus and pneumonia or pleurisy, these did not include any of the acute infectious diseases that had commanded so much attention among contemporaries.

One may summarise the 'killers' of male adults in 1913 as follows:

(1) The percentage of unspecified or unknown causes of death had fallen sharply; overall figures seem to have become more reliable than they were in 1876.

(2) As before, the most important was pulmonary tuberculosis, which accounted for 18.3 per cent of all deaths, followed by heart and circulatory disorders, which killed 14.3 per cent.

(3) If pneumonia and the other pulmonary diseases are added to tuberculosis, the percentage of deaths from diseases of the respiratory organs amounted to more than 33 per cent. Compared with the figures for 1876, however, this was a decline of between 10 and 12 percentage points.

(4) By 1913, the relative numbers of deaths caused by cancer (8.3 per cent) and nervous disorders (5.4 per cent) had increased considerably, a reason for this no doubt being that they were more accurately diagnosed than before. The proportion of other digestive disorders (other than vomiting and diarrhoea, etc.) had increased slightly.

(5) All of the named infectious diseases — apart from the contagious animal diseases, tuberculosis and other diseases of the respiratory organs (i.e. scarlet fever, measles, German measles, diphtheria, croup, whooping-cough, typhus, erysypelas, other infections from wounds, influenza and 'other contagious diseases') — accounted for no more than a total of 2.4 per cent of all deaths in Prussian adult males aged between 30 and 60.

Obviously, the pattern of causes of death among this age group did not change in any fundamental way between 1876 and 1913, though a few marginal shifts did take place. Noticeable developments were the decline in mortality from tuberculosis, which was partially, if not totally, compensated for by the increase in other diseases of the respiratory organs, and the fall in the cases of typhus and unspecified or unknown illnesses. At the same time, though, there was after the turn of the century a steady rise in the percentage of deaths caused by cardiac or circulatory diseases, cancer and diseases of the nervous system.

In a further part of my investigation, the results of which will not be documented here, mortality rates in Prussia in the sample years 1876, 1901, 1903 and 1913 were analysed by age and by cause of death in more detail. Particular emphasis was placed on calculating regional deviations from the Prussian average which could be attributed to structural socio-economic differences.[26] This analysis highlighted even more clearly the manner in which the pattern of causes of death was changing, which has been discussed above. The fact that tuberculosis was by far the most significant cause of death for those over 15 years of age is most interesting. Moreover, it is evident that this was not a disease (or cause of death) which was more prominent among the urban working population. It can be regarded as the bane of the lower classes in both town and country. The Prussian regions with above-average mortality rates among adults were those which were most heavily industrialised (here in the late nineteenth century the secondary sector was expanding particularly quickly). This pattern was even more pronounced in the older age groups. As might be expected, the number of men over 40 or 50, especially in industrial regions, who died of tuberculosis, other respiratory diseases or accidents, was higher than the Prussian average. The high incidence of tuberculosis and cardiac and circulatory diseases among these men indicates that they were exposed to excessive work loads and long-term physical wear and tear, and the other major causes of death (other respiratory diseases, accidents) point to the damaging effect of working conditions — for example heavy exposure to gases, dust, dirt, and so on — on their health.

The general trends revealed by this analysis can be summed up relatively simply. Men over 40 paid the price of industrialisation, higher productivity and better opportunities for those living in

---

26. See Spree, 'Volksgesundheit'; idem, 'Veränderungen des Todesursachen-Panoramas'.

urban and industrial environments. Above all, the health of children, young men and women of child-bearing age benefited from life in the towns. There were signs as early as the end of the nineteenth century that the population pyramid was gradually becoming 'top heavy', with the older age groups in particular comprising more and more women who had outlived their male counterparts. On the other hand, as a result of the changes in the pattern of causes of death we have been discussing, the various regions became more alike with respect to the range of mortality rates among all age groups.

1.5 Summary: Changing Trends in the 'People's Health'

The increase in life expectancy in the period under discussion, combined with the fall in the average mortality rate, creates the impression that, far from worsening, the level of the 'people's health' had probably begun to improve by the mid-1880s at the latest. However, this view appears to be undermined by the few direct indicators of the overall health situation that are available: the frequency and duration of the illnesses suffered by the members of statutory sickness insurance funds. The national average number of working days lost per member rose from 6.1 per annum in 1885 to 7.0 in 1903 and to 8.7 in 1913.[27] This corresponds to an increase of 2.6 days in the frequency of sickness. At the same time, the average number of working days lost for each case of illness (an indication of the duration of an illness) rose by an average of 6.6 days from 14.0 in 1885 to 20.6 in 1913. Finally, the number of days spent in hospital care could also be regarded with some justification as an indicator of a fall in the overall level of health, since it increased almost threefold between 1877 and 1901 and then over the next ten years by two-thirds of the previous growth rate.[28] This suggests that, at the turn of the century, the annual number of days spent in hospital care accelerated at a rate that was more than three times the population growth rate between 1877 and 1913. However, one should resist the temptation to interpret these figures as a reflection of a real increase in the threat posed by sickness. What happened was that as people perceived some form of ailment they began to

---

27. Calculated from *Statistisches Jahrbuch für das Deutsche Reich*, vol. 8 (1887), and vol. 36 (1915).
28. See P. vor dem Esche, 'Die Versorgung der Bevölkerung mit Krankenhäusern in Deutschland von 1876 bis zur Gegenwart', *Archiv für Hygiene*, *138* (1954), p. 397.

make more frequent and widespread use of the opportunity to undergo hospital treatment. They were no doubt encouraged in this by the statutory sickness insurance, on the one hand, and the growing prestige of hospital medicine, on the other.

At this point, we should clarify some of the main trends evident in the information presented above:

(1) The decline in the average mortality rate affected all age groups, with the exception of infants, from the mid-1880s at the latest. In general, this decline also applied to all the different regions and sizes of population involved, though in certain cases the rate fell more slowly than the national average. In the Eastern provinces of Prussia, and even in some of the heavily industrialised areas in the West, the fall in the mortality rate was both slower and less marked until well into the twentieth century and in some cases even into the 1920s. The same applied to adults in the cities who were aged 30 or more. Conversely, though, in view of the disproportionately sharp decline in mortality in the various age groups, the living standards and health of young city-dwellers would seem to have improved. Initially this applied to the 15–30 age groups, but then extended to all the younger age groups, and gradually they began to enjoy greater and greater advantages over their counterparts in rural areas.

(2) The analysis of the pattern of causes of death showed that a number of marked changes had taken place during the period under investigation which also seem to point to certain developments in the level of the 'people's health'. One particularly interesting finding concerned the incidence of death from tuberculosis, which declined steadily throughout the period. The effect this had on the overall standard of health was by no means cancelled out by the temporary increase in the other infections of the respiratory organs. Nevertheless, on the national level, diseases of the respiratory organs remained the most common cause of death in all regions and in every age group from the age of 15 upwards. A comparison of the relative number of deaths caused by tuberculosis in several different regions showed that by 1913 there was less variation in regional levels (though they had not evened out completely), and that the differences between the agricultural and the highly industrial areas had continued to shrink. In the light of this, the view that tuberculosis was the typical disease of the urban industrial worker is simply untenable.

(3) In general terms, the changes in the pattern of causes of death were shaped by a fall in the number of cases of acute infectious diseases to which young people in particular were prone, and

which often resulted in death after a very short time. There were, however, a number of infectious diseases that did not conform to this pattern — for example, other diseases of the respiratory organs, which were fatal predominantly among the middle-aged or elderly. These age groups were also hit by increased mortality from coronary or circulatory disease, cancer and diseases of the stomach, intestines and nervous system. The greater frequency of these diseases may be interpreted as signs of physical reactions to the cumulative disorders associated in particular with occupations which in the long term placed great strains on the individual's physical and nervous condition. This would not only explain why they were fatal only in the older age groups. It would also account for the fact that although there were no significant regional differences in the percentages of deaths caused by tuberculosis or coronary and circulatory diseases in the 30–60 age group, in the 60–70 age group of 1913 in the highly industrialised Western administrative districts of Prussia, relatively more people were dying from these two diseases than in the Eastern provinces.

(4) On balance, I would conclude that it is not possible to speak of an overall improvement in the level of the 'people's health' in this particular period. Children and teenagers — and perhaps even adults up to the age of 30 — benefited from a fall in the mortality rate, and thus could expect to live longer. It is also highly probable that they became less susceptible to the most serious causes of death in the late nineteenth century, which, in these age groups, became increasingly less common in the years before 1914 (with regard to both the level of mortality in each age group and the percentage of deaths they caused in each age group). The health of adults over the age of 30, on the other hand, seems to have been affected by a number of contradictory developments. The fall in the average mortality rates in these age groups may well have been accompanied by increased morbidity, cumulative ill-health, signs of physical wear and tear and a gradual weakening of immunity to disease. Generally speaking, such developments may take several decades before becoming fatal, but they may still have been the reason for the growing number of men and women who suffered at a premature stage from some form of inability to work, invalidity or long-term illness.

(5) If we are correct in assuming that changes in the pattern of causes of death can serve as an indicator of levels of health, then it can be said that various social groups, divided according to the nature of their ability to work, or more exactly according to the particular conditions and strains associated with their work, would

have been affected in different ways by these changes. The more severe the physical stresses and strains or the effects of noise, dirt, cold, damp and dust at the workplace, the more likely it is that the health of the individual would be prematurely impaired. It should be remembered, however, that this would not necessarily have caused mortality in the occupational group in question to rise. Consequently, it can also be assumed that as these sorts of working conditions become more common, so data on mortality become a less suitable measurement of the 'people's health'. In terms of the theoretical framework of social inequality outlined above, this means that statistical analyses of causes of death are not sufficiently sophisticated to yield information on how the predominant working conditions typical for the acquisition classes translate low market capacities (low and unspecific levels of qualification) into long-term and chronic detrimental effects on health. Such effects can be interpreted as factors occasioning an additional reduction in workers' market capacity in the second half of their lives, and can be regarded as typical examples of intra-generational social decline. Perhaps this kind of process might explain the decline in wages which, as Borscheid and Schomerus show,[29] is characteristic of industrial workers after the age of 30 or, at the latest, 40.

(6) Since we are concerned here with examining changes in the general level of health, it must be remembered that, from the beginning of the twentieth century at the latest, the German economy was becoming progressively more industrialised, with the effect that the relative number of occupations associated with the unfavourable conditions described above was declining at an increasing rate. On the other hand, in the wake of mechanisation and rationalisation, stress as a factor impairing health became more significant in the long term. The conclusion must be that the absolute number of people suffering from chronic illnesses, premature invalidity or prolonged sickness had increased by the end of the period under investigation. But this was not because the living and working conditions of sections of the working class had worsened. It was rather the case that changes in the pattern of causes of death led to an increase in the number of older workers, and thus in the reservoir of people susceptible to chronic, nervous and longer-term ailments. But it is exactly because of this absolute growth in the number of older people that, contrary to what is

---

29. See P. Borscheid and H. Schomerus, 'Mobilität und soziale Lage der württembergischen Fabrikarbeiterschaft im 19. Jahrhundert' in P.J. Müller (ed.), *Die Analyse prozeß-produzierter Daten* (vol. 2 of Historisch-sozialwissenschaftliche Forschungen) (Stuttgart, 1977), pp. 205–11.

occasionally claimed, it is unlikely that there was an increase in the *percentage* of those over 30 or 40 suffering from premature invalidity, long-term illnesses, chronic diseases and so forth.

(7) As far as health as a resource (in terms of market capacity) is concerned, the difference between town and country gradually became less significant as an element of class formation. The reason was that the adverse effects of working and living conditions in the urban industrial areas became less pronounced than they had been when compared to the situation in agriculture — at least for the under-40s.

As was shown above, the quality of the available data means that we can only draw essentially indirect conclusions about the social inequalities affecting health and morbidity. More precisely, although a large amount of information on the effects of social differences on health is available — particularly with regard to mortality — it was almost exclusively gathered for a specific point in time, generally applies to narrowly defined geographical areas and, as a rule, was obtained by using non-comparable differential criteria. It is therefore impossible to chart any clear developments or patterns from the existing mass of relevant data. On the contrary, we tend to arrive at a diversified collection of information which creates a distinctly static impression: death was more common and came at an earlier age among those who were poor, lived in cramped housing with poor sanitation, worked in insecure jobs which they frequently had to change, or had learnt no useful skill or trade. In other words, merely individual aspects of the poverty syndrome are obtained, which have not been welded together into any form of structured context that might help us to identify the first signs of historical changes. There are, however, a few exceptions to this, in the form of studies which analyse inequality from what is termed an indirect or ecological perspective, in which regional units, rather than individuals, are the bearers of particular characteristics. However, the conclusions that may be drawn from this kind of approach, especially as far as mortality rates are concerned, are extremely unreliable — all the more so when longer periods of time are involved.

One example of an ecological approach which also includes a long-term comparison is a study of the mortality rates in the city of Bremen between 1876 and 1900 that was based on a comparative study of a number of socio-economically distinguishable urban residential areas (or streets).[30] The most important conclusion to be

30. See J. Funk, 'Die Sterblichkeit nach sozialen Klassen in der Stadt Bremen', *Mitteilungen des Bremischen Statistischen Amtes im Jahre 1911*, no. 1 (Bremen, 1911), pp. 1–12.

drawn is that the differences between the average mortality rates of the various urban areas clearly increased during the period under discussion. The better the residential area, the greater was the fall in the mortality rate, which in turn resulted in an increase in the regional differences. However, such a thesis should first be tested by examining the changes in the composition of the residential population by age and social group. Unless this is done, it can only apply to the specific areas themselves rather than the actual groups of people resident in them. Moreover, one should not be tempted to make an automatic causal connection between the quality of housing and life chances from this example alone, because it may well have been the case that ill-health and loss of income had forced people to move to cheaper housing with correspondingly inadequate hygiene standards.[31] Those suffering from chronic diseases tended to be concentrated in areas with cheaper housing. This seems to be additional evidence of the process of collective social decline mentioned above, which characterised the lives of large sections of the working class in this period and which was a result of working under conditions damaging to health.

The number of deaths from tuberculosis is a further indicator of the unequal distribution of life chances — in other words of different market capacities and the way they changed. In Prussia the average number of deaths from TB among the total population fell by 38 per cent between 1875 and 1903, the fall accelerating further up to 1913 (319 deaths per 100,000 inhabitants in 1875, 197 in 1903, 137 in 1913).[32] If the rates for urban and rural communities are compared, it becomes clear that throughout this period the TB mortality rate was higher in the towns than in the country, that it fell more slowly in the towns and that consequently the percentage difference between these two rates actually increased from 26 per cent in 1876 to 35 per cent in 1914.[33]

---

31. This is a factor which is typical even today when slums are created. On such consequences of TB see inter alia D. Blasius, 'Geschichte und Krankheit. Sozialgeschichtliche Perspektiven der Medizingeschichte', *Geschichte und Gesellschaft*, 2 (3) (1976), pp. 397–402; A. Grotjahn, *Soziale Pathologie*, 3rd edn (Berlin, 1923), pp. 51–64 and 70–5.

32. See A. Kayserling, 'Die Tuberkulose in ihrem Verhältnis zur Mortalität in Deutschland' in B. Fränkel (ed.), *Der Stand der Tuberkulose-Bekämpfung in Deutschland. Denkschrift, dem Internationalen Tuberkulose-Kongreß in Paris 1905* (Berlin, 1905), pp. 8–9; Grotjahn, *Soziale Pathologie*, p. 49.

33. This result must be partly due to the problem of defining the town. An investigation into the decline in mortality from TB between 1886–8 and 1903–5 at the level of Prussian administrative districts showed that on the whole the declines in the more industrialised, populated and urbanised western districts were considerably larger than those in the eastern districts, which were all below the average; see Hillenberg, quoted in Grotjahn, *Soziale Pathologie*, p. 68.

In addition to variations in the fall of TB mortality according to region and size of community, the different ways in which the sexes and various age groups were affected were equally important. The discrepancy between the sexes is demonstrated by the fact that at the beginning of the period under discussion, women in Prussia were on average less likely to die from tuberculosis than men. By the turn of the century the advantages women enjoyed had been considerably eroded: the excess mortality rate for men fell from 25 per cent (355 men to 283 women per 100,000 inhabitants in 1875) to 19 per cent (207 to 174 in 1902). By 1913 it had fallen to as low as 8 per cent (142 to 131).[34] A more detailed breakdown by age of the TB mortality rate among women shows that it fell by no more than a minimal amount between 1875–9 and 1914 in the 20–40 age group.[35] The rate for females was slightly higher than for males from the age of five upwards. In 1875–9 it was higher only in the under-20s, but by 1901 it remained higher up to the age of 30, and after 1911 up to 40. If this relative deterioration in the health of women of working age is a reflection of the consequences of more women finding employment in urban and industrial environments (and for the majority of working-class women this meant the double burden of domestic housework and outside employment), then it is a further example of the way social class functions as a mechanism affecting health.

From the 1890s onwards, the significance of this dimension was repeatedly documented by the emerging disciplines of occupational and industrial health, though unfortunately the information available is restricted to specific times and places, and is therefore not suitable for comparative study. One particularly detailed study of the city of Stuttgart between 1893 and 1902 divided the population into three social groups according to occupational position (putting the self-employed, those in the liberal professions and senior public officials in one group, middle and junior public officials and white-collar workers in the second, and blue-collar workers, servants and casual labourers in the third). The actual TB mortality rate of each group (subdivided by age) was compared with the expected rate of each group calculated from the percentage of the population

---

34. From A. Würzburg, 'Über den Einfluß des Alters und des Geschlechts auf Sterblichkeit an Lungenschwindsucht', *Mitteilungen aus dem Kaiserlichen Gesundheitsamte* vol. 2 (Berlin, 1884), pp. 96–7; Keyserling, 'Die Tuberkulose', pp. 8–9; Grotjahn, *Soziale Pathologie*, p. 50.
35. From Würzburg, 'Über den Einfluß', pp. 96–7; *Das Gesundheitswesen des Preußischen Staates im Jahre 1901* (Berlin, 1903), p. 221; B. Möllers, 'Deutsche Tuberkulosestatistik' in K.H. Blümel (ed.), *Handbuch der Tuberkulose-Fürsorge* (Munich, 1926), vol. 1, pp. 157–8.

involved.[36] In all age groups (from 20 to 69) the actual TB rate in the working class was higher than the expected rate and exceeded the rates in both of the other groups by a considerable amount — in fact, on average by almost 80 per cent. These data lend support to the thesis, which, although extremely general, does seem to be highly convincing given the vast amount of heterogeneous material, that even as late as the last years of the Wilhelmine Empire the working class (in the broadest sense) must be regarded as a deprived group in terms of health-dependent and health-determined market capacity, whereas public officials and white-collar workers in particular and some of the self-employed seem to have been privileged. As we have already mentioned, it is important to remember in this context that relatively poor health can be a consequence of low market capacity, and that, conversely, if health begins to be impaired (especially by chronic diseases), the market capacity of individuals or groups can be reduced even further.

In the context of this book, the arguments outlined above are important because they help us to define the framework within which it is possible meaningfully to interpret the relationship between structured social inequality and illness and death. At the same time though, the conclusions we have been able to draw thus far have remained rather vague, because they have generally been based on rather indirect evidence. In the following chapter we shall examine health and illness as they affected one specific age group (in this case infants) so as to be able to establish with a considerable degree of precision the connection between the 'causal components of market situation' (socio-structural features), on the one hand, and the infant mortality rate, on the other, partly by introducing a number of indicators reflecting particular life styles.

36. See W. Weinberg, 'Die Tuberkulose in Stuttgart 1873–1902', *Medicinisches Correspondenz-Blatt des württembergischen ärztlichen Landesvereins*, 76 (1906), pp. 25–6.

2
Infant Mortality as a Mirror of Social Inequality

2.1 Infant Mortality as an Indicator: Concepts and Sources

The considerable regional variations in the levels of infant mortality in Germany had aroused the attention of demographers and statisticians as early as the first half of the nineteenth century.[37] Climatic, ethnic, biological (racial, for example) and geographical factors were cited as the hypothetical causes of these differences.[38] But even at an early stage, it was recognised that these factors probably only affected infant mortality rates in some socially mediated form — that is, when enmeshed with certain socio-cultural values and attitudes, and in the economic structures and behavioural patterns associated with them.[39] From the last third of the nineteenth century up until the First World War, there was a rapid growth in

---

37. Infant mortality is defined here as the percentage of infants up to the age of 12 full months who died during the calendar year compared with all living births of the same period. This definition is somewhat imprecise since the number of deaths is not compared to the age cohort from which the deaths resulted. If groups are compared over a long period, the results are not affected by any distortion which might be caused by this method. Rahts's correction formula is not applied because it would only improve the applicability of a particular figure to a particular year, which is irrelevant in our case. Still-births are not included in the calculations. Since almost all analysed data refer to Prussia, there is no danger that excluding still-births introduces any errors into comparisons between states. Births and deaths of legitimate and illegitimate infants are included unless specifically stated otherwise. Since we are concerned with the social inequalities of social groups in the face of death, limiting the investigation exclusively to legitimate infants would be unjustified because the respective proportion of illegitimate births is one of the features typical of the various social groups we are examining. In addition, the widely varying occurrence of post-nuptial legitimation of illegitimate offspring in different groups would considerably complicate the calculations.

38. See the regional infant mortality rates in the nineteenth and early twentieth centuries in J.E. Knodel, *The Decline of Fertility in Germany 1871–1939* (Princeton, NJ, 1974), pp. 170 and 186; F. Prinzing, 'Die Entwickelung der Kindersterblichkeit in den europäischen Staaten', *Jahrbücher für Nationalökonomie und Statistik*, third series, 17 (1899), pp. 577–635; idem, *Handbuch*, 2nd edn, pp. 373–81. Noteworthy also for its 'modern' findings is E. Roesle, 'Die Sterblichkeit im ersten Lebensmonat. Ein internationaler, statistischer Vergleich', *Zeitschrift für soziale Medizin*, 5 (1910), pp. 151–212.

39. See *inter alia* K. Seutemann, *Kindersterblichkeit sozialer Bevölkerungsgruppen insbesondere im preußischen Staate und seinen Provinzen* (Tübingen, 1894), pp. 7–10,

the number of attempts to investigate the factors affecting infant mortality on an empirical and statistical basis. Some of these studies recognised such mediators as intervening variables. The factors which deserve particular attention are those which still serve as points of reference in more recent studies of infant mortality — for example sex, legitimacy, the contrast between town and country, parental occupation, wealth, housing conditions and dietary patterns. Moreover, the importance of the age of the mother, her occupation and the specific demands placed on her at work, the influence of family size, and the number and frequency of births have long been recognised as significant.

We have thus listed the most important criteria that can be used to interpret and differentiate levels of infant mortality. However, even in more recent studies, it is only rarely that we find a clear conceptual framework specifying the relations between them or the extent to which they mutually compensate or reinforce any given effects. The few studies that have attempted to classify this set of variables and test them for systematic connections are the exceptions.

This even applies to those cases where the material under analysis was obtained and processed on the basis of suitably formulated questionnaires. In this respect present-day socio-historical and socio-demographic research, like older, contemporary studies, is always obliged to rely on the second-hand analysis of data collected in a number of different ways using a whole range of different types of question, and is thus faced with a task which from the outset can produce only inadequate results.

In the following, I shall outline a theoretical model composed of two levels which will provide the point of departure for the interpretation below of the infant mortality indicator. The variations in the infant-mortality rate will be interpreted as a reflection of the structures of social inequality that shape the way infants and young children are cared for and brought up. This inequality is a result both of the material conditions and environment surrounding the process of care, and of the attitudes and behavioural charac-

---

157–64; Prinzing, *Handbuch*, 2nd edn, pp. 384–5. A recent and comprehensive account is given by H.J. Kintner, 'The Determinants of Infant Mortality in Germany from 1871 to 1933' (PhD thesis, University of Michigan, 1982). A.E. Imhof attempts to explain the variation in infant mortality rates in 'Unterschiedliche Säuglingssterblichkeit in Deutschland, 18. bis 20. Jahrhundert — Warum?', *Zeitschrift für Bevölkerungswissenschaft*, 7 (3) (1981), pp. 343–82. Finally, see R.W. Lee, 'Regional Differences in the Population Growth of Germany in the Early 19th Century' in R. Fremdling and R.H. Tilly (eds), *Industrialisierung und Raum. Studien zur regionalen Differenzierung im Deutschland des 19. Jahrhunderts* (Stuttgart, 1979).

teristics of the people dispensing that care. Bronfenbrenner makes an initial attempt at structuring this complex web of influences in abstract terms, and defines a number of 'parameters of the social ecology of human development'[40] which form three overlapping and increasingly more general levels:

(1) The immediate material, spatial and social environment of each child, which is created by the child itself and by the people participating directly in the process of care.

(2) The superimposed level of material, and above all social, institutions i.e. the various actual environments (such as urban district or community), social networks (such as informal social groups, family, peer groups, circles of friends and neighbours) and the formalised and organised systems of roles associated with elements of the infrastructure such as the health service, education and the social services.

(3) In so far as it contributes to the structuring of the process of socialisation and care, the ideological system which furnishes the social networks, institutions, roles and activities of the two previous levels with motives and meanings.

It is clear that the 'parameters of social ecology' refer to the various analytical dimensions of the material, social and ideological conditions of care and upbringing that are shaped by social inequality. They may serve as the basis for a discussion that will lead to the formulation of a theoretical framework which is both more concrete and more suitable for a socio-historical approach. Because my own work avoids concentrating on individual (i.e. biographical) cases, in the following I shall have to forgo all attempts to identify precisely the individual variables on the 'motive level' and to establish relevant indicators. Since it is not possible to observe or quantify past actions or patterns of behaviour at first hand, in naming three relatively general sets of behavioural variables affecting the care of infants and young children, I am fully aware that without exception the indicators relating to them can only provide indirect information about the actual, historical processes of care and the behaviour which accompanied them. A matrix of variables that hopes to reflect the complexity of the subject should refer to: the direct forms of care (the specific features of the way each social group behaves with regard to the care of infants and young children); the typical patterns of interaction and the living conditions of the family, household and neighbourhood (to the extent that they are relevant to care); and consumer behaviour and leisure activities.

40. U. Bronfenbrenner, *Ökologische Sozialisationsforschung* (Stuttgart, 1976), p. 203.

However, the set of indicators that can be derived from such a matrix is still far too extensive. I thus intend to deal with no more than a few of all the possible indicators, and even these will not always be treated in a systematic context. I shall concentrate on diet and nutritional methods, family size and, on occasion, on the quality of housing. Although these indicators are not always entirely reliable and considerable reservations remain, they none the less allow us to make certain inferences about the conditions and forms associated with the care of infants and the level of its success, especially in the specific historical situation we are examining here. They are defined on an intermediate level between class formation and social stratification.

A particular set of indicators can prove to be meaningful and useful only if related to a variable. For our period, I regard this to be the differential infant mortality rate which, in my view, also functions as an indicator of important dimensions of the life chances associated with a given social milieu. The approach I have adopted is deliberate in that it pays heed to the prevalent preoccupations of the socio-political debates of the day and, more particularly, of the literature of the time on social medicine and public health.[41] It is clear that in choosing the indicators of varying conditions of care, I have ensured that they are demonstrably linked to infant mortality. For although the latter measures the success of care — which varies according to socio-structural and socio-cultural determinants — from a negative perspective (i.e. it records above all the failure of that care), it nevertheless expresses the way a number of casual influences can combine to affect an individual's market capacity. In other words, it provides information on the distribution of life chances.

Perhaps it would be helpful to list more schematically the factors directly or indirectly affecting the level of infant mortality. In order to do this, I have adopted an approach that is related directly to the individual. Accordingly, the contention here is that the infant mortality rate seems to depend primarily on three factors: on the extent of pre-natal damage; on the extent to which the infant is

---

41. Typical examples are: G. Tugendreich, 'Der Einfluß der sozialen Lage auf Krankheit und Sterblichkeit des Kindes' in M. Mosse and G. Tugendreich (eds), *Krankheit und soziale Lage* (Munich, 1913), pp. 266ff and 304; M Baum, 'Grundriß der Säuglingsfürsorge' in S. Engel, *Grundriß der Säuglingskunde*, 10th edn (Munich, 1920), pp. 189ff. For modern interpretations see United Nations Department of Social Affairs, Population Division, *Foetal, Infant and Early Childhood Mortality, vol. 2: Biological, Social and Economic Factors, Population Studies, 13* (1954); H.G. Birch and J.D. Gussow, *Disadvantaged Children. Health, Nutrition and School Failure* (New York and London, 1970), esp. pp. 12–13 and 266ff.

exposed to infection or, alternatively, on his or her physical ability to resist disease and remain immune to infection; and finally on the extent to which care is not provided (for example, if the child is totally neglected, is a victim of malnutrition, does not have adequate clothing, etc.). Factors indirectly determining the level of infant mortality include: the quality of housing (especially with regard to hygiene); the quality of diet; and the standard of personal hygiene, clothing and supervision. These factors primarily affect the degree to which the child is exposed to — and its ability to resist — disease. The quality of the child's diet is particularly important in this respect (and this includes the provision of relatively regular meals, which might also come under the category of 'quality of care'), because during the period we are investigating, a clear distinction was made between 'artificial feeding' (*künstliche Ernährung*) and 'breast-feeding by mothers' (*Selbst-Stillen*) in discussions on how dietary standards might help to reduce the infant mortality rate.

There is another consideration. The determinants mentioned above also point to the most important components of market capacity: the occupation and income of the parents. However, these are related to particular traditions and skills in the care and upbringing of children — that is, to components of social stratification. Finally, there is a close interrelationship between the occupation and income of the parents and the particular socio-cultural tradition of child care, on the one hand, and the age at which people marry, the level of fertility, the frequency of births and the average family size, on the other. It must be noted, however, that the way in which such interrelationships operate in each case is often difficult to explain. Even the health of the parents can come into play.

Before presenting the empirical findings, I would like to elaborate briefly on the origin and quality of the source material on feeding methods and levels of infant mortality. I have only used figures taken from published data. One source is official statistical surveys. The official data (*Preußische Statistik*) have been particularly useful, since, from 1877 onwards, births, marriages and deaths were classified according to social position (of the father if the parents were married and of the mother if they were not), which renders the data suitable for analysis. After 1902, the categories of social position were brought into line with those that had been used by the Imperial Occupational Census since 1895, and this markedly improved their clarity and depth of focus. From the end of the 1800s, similar data also began to be published by the Statistical Office of the State of Saxony. In addition, a number of individual

Statistical Offices collected data showing that the infant mortality rate varied according to the social group involved.[42]

Official surveys, which testify to the efforts by the authorities to record differences in infant mortality rates and their causes, can all be traced back to the public discussion and campaign which focused on the conditions affecting infant mortality and how it could be reduced. These also gave rise to the second type of source we are able to draw on: surveys conducted by committed private individuals and, more importantly, by private organisations. Such people and organisations became heavily involved in a campaign which, after the turn of the century, developed into a large-scale middle-class movement to combat infant mortality, especially among the lower classes. Such surveys were often based on interviews with midwives, although they were sometimes conducted by medical officials (for example, they made comprehensive surveys of specific administrative districts or towns). The results were occasionally published as monographs, but more usually as articles in journals dealing with medicine, public health, and social policy. Unfortunately, however, these older publications, whether official or private, often have serious shortcomings which render the data more or less useless, at least as far as infant mortality rates are concerned. For example, population samples are ill-defined, the number of deaths rather than mortality rates are given. Thus whilst these surveys do contain a wealth of information, very little of it can be utilised in any systematic statistical analysis.

2.2 Infant Mortality and Parental Wealth

For a long time it was considered that a general measure of prosperity could be derived from socially differentiated infant mortality rates. Concomitantly, statistical material was collected in such a way that various regions (mostly urban districts and streets) were ranked according to an index of prosperity, and then related to the respective levels of infant mortality. In these calculations, the ecological approach was adopted and the most varied criteria were taken as indicators of social status. Elsewhere I have presented three contrasting examples illustrating different techniques of measurement and their possible implications (relating to Leipzig in 1875; Frankfurt am Main in 1870–80; and Munich in 1902–7).[43] The

---

42. For an overview see Prinzing, *Handbuch*, 2nd edn, chapter 4; G. Tugendreich, *Die Mutter- und Säuglingsfürsorge* (Stuttgart, 1910), pp. 54–81.
43. See Spree, 'Strukturierte soziale Ungleichheit', Tables 1–3, pp. 69–70. For

results tend to be the same: the infant mortality rate falls as wealth increases. Since the data analysed were obtained from different regions (towns) and recorded at different times, and since, moreover, the subjects under investigation (the urban districts and streets) were not identical, it does not seem possible to compare the various mortality rates directly. I shall therefore not attempt to present the data. However, the situation is different for the disparity between the lowest and the highest infant mortality rates. In each of the examples, the range between these two extremes varies considerably, depending on the feature deemed to define social status. The range was smallest in Frankfurt, where the number of households with servants per urban district was selected as the differential criterion. The figure here was some 13 per cent, which means that the excess mortality rate in the most deprived area was 183 per cent compared with mortality in the most privileged area. The range was greatest in Leipzig, where the criterion was taken to be the number of people per room. Here the figure was more than 30 per cent, which corresponds to an excess mortality rate of 377 per cent in the streets with overcrowded housing.

A further example of the putative connection between parental wealth and the level of infant mortality is shown in Table 3. It shows the results of calculations made to establish the strength of the relationship between the infant mortality rate and the relative prosperity of each district in the city of Berlin in three years between 1886 and 1910. The advantage Table 3 has over the examples referred to above is that it allows us to follow developments over an extended period. The method of calculation and the index used to measure wealth are explained in the notes to the table, so I shall restrict myself here to an interpretation of the results. If we begin by concentrating on the correlation coefficients shown in the first line, it is apparent that in 1886, as expected, the level of infant mortality was clearly inversely proportional to the level of prosperity in each urban district. By the outbreak of the First World War, the relationship was only slightly less pronounced. A further trend may be deduced from the fourth line of Table 3 which shows the excess mortality rates obtained by expressing the highest

---

further examples see K. Freudenberg, 'Fruchtbarkeit und Sterblichkeit in den Berliner Verwaltungsbezirken in Beziehung zu deren sozialer Struktur' in A. Grotjahn et al. (eds), *Ergebnisse der sozialen Hygiene und Gesundheitsfürsorge* (Leipzig, 1929), vol. 1; E.G. Stockwell, 'Infant Mortality and Socio-Economic Status; A Changing Relationship', *Milbank Memorial Fund Quarterly*, 40 (1962), pp. 105ff; C. V. Willie, 'A Research Note on the Changing Association between Infant Mortality and Socio-Economic Status', *Social Forces*, 37 (1958–9), pp. 225ff; For an overview see also Seutemann's introduction; Prinzing, *Handbuch*, 1st edn, pp. 300–4.

mortality rate as a percentage of the lowest. It seems that social inequality actually increased in the years before the turn of the century, only to decline again marginally between 1900 and 1910.

If we recall the discussion above on the set of determinants of the level of infant mortality, the differences in the excess mortality rates revealed in the examples cited are understandable. The number of households with servants is a relatively superficial consideration compared with factors which directly affect mortality levels, and cannot even be regarded as a reliable yardstick of parental income or occupational position. The average rent, on the other hand, which proved to be the most important differential criterion in the Munich example, gives a much clearer picture — though one that is still comparatively general — of the level of resources which may have been expended on infant care. Even here though, the relationship is an indirect one. Infant care, and the nature of the conditions surrounding it, are most directly affected by the number of people living in each room. This was the differential criterion used in the Berlin and Leipzig examples (see Table 3). The degree of overcrowding that is reflected in the increase in the number of inhabitants per room is directly related to the likelihood of exposure to infectious diseases, quite apart from the fact that it also probably leads to an accumulation of other factors impairing the health of infants. The fourfold rise in the infant mortality rate in Leipzig when overcrowding increased would suggest this. The fact that the difference between the highest and lowest mortality rates in Table 3 is considerably smaller than 400 per cent, is undoubtedly a consequence of the fact that the urban districts in the Berlin example were much less homogeneous than the residential streets of Leipzig. (This illustrates a problem which often arises when social inequality is measured by indirect means. A relatively large body of information on the social composition of the formal units must be available before one can judge how homogeneous they are in relation to the subject under analysis. However, attempts to create a certain level of homogeneity tend to be hampered at an early stage because there is a lack of individual data that can be used as a starting point.)

The examples that have been discussed here remain problematic, however, because the information they provide on the causal components of market capacity and, equally, on the components of social stratification is inadequate. Any inferences that may be drawn concerning the relationship between the causal components and the level of infant mortality must therefore be regarded as extremely questionable. Thus the following section shall attempt to consider other, more reliable indicators of social inequality.

2.3 Infant Mortality and Parental Occupation

The conceptualisation of social inequality discussed above made it clear that it is impossible in theory to determine either the class position or the social status of the individual with any reliability on the basis of a single indicator. Class formation and social stratification are multi-dimensional processes which can only be adequately understood by using different indicators to measure the various major dimensions. None the less, in practice, historians and sociologists — influenced by the gaps in the information at their disposal and by their limited time and energy — have tended to subscribe to the opinion that the best single indicator of 'the overall position of an individual in the system of stratification in industrialised societies' is membership of a particular occupational group.[44] Other resources determining the market capacity of an individual — especially income, health, education, social status and political power — are intimately bound up with membership of an occupational group, and are even sometimes seen as being largely determined by it. It can scarcely be denied that there is a close link between occupation and other marketable resources, and there can be no doubt that the latter do greatly affect access to the former. Obviously a kind of dialectical relationship exists that cannot be broken down conclusively at the level of indicators (criteria of analysis). For there is no single and unambiguous pattern to the way in which social factors determine, and are determined by, other factors, nor is it possible in principle to divide the factors involved into dependent and independent variables. This is precisely one of the things the framework outlined above is intended to show. None the less, it may be argued that at the level of the individual, his or her occupation is a reliable indicator of his or her market capacity at a given point in time. Unfortunately, in the following it will generally not be possible to refer to occupation as a criterion of analysis, but only to what may be termed 'occupational status'. In more precise terms, this refers to a combination of several items of information which, in most cases, can actually be interpreted as an expression of market capacity, and which simultaneously includes aspects of the attribution of social status — that is, aspects of social stratification.

The most detailed and chronologically the most extensive material which can be evaluated from this particular perspective is that

---

44. J. Kocka, 'Theorien in der Sozial- und Gesellschaftsgeschichte. Vorschläge zur historischen Schichtungsanalyse', *Geschichte und Gesellschaft*, *1* (1) (1975), p. 41.

which was produced by official statisticians in Prussia, the largest German state in existence during the period under investigation. From 1877 onwards, the Prussian Statistical Office published the annual number of births and deaths classified according to both occupational group (of the father where the parents were married and of the mother when they were not) and occupational status. The criteria of occupational status were the (presumed) permanence of occupation, and the somewhat more problematic distinction between dependent wage-earners and self-employed. Up to 1901 occupational status was not further subdivided into the more important economic sectors. Individuals were classified according to occupational status, on the one hand, and occupational group or economic sector on the other, these two categories being recorded separately, but aggregated, with the result that they cannot be combined retrospectively. From 1902 onwards, the two criteria were combined. From this point it becomes possible to compare, for example, the levels of infant mortality among white- and blue-collar workers in different branches of the economy. Since, however, the emphasis here is on the long-term comparison, the more detailed subdivisions dating from 1902 have had to take second place. The attempt has been made to keep valid until 1913 the rather approximate subdivisions that had been used from the late nineteenth century onwards. For some years, comparative material from other German states has also been included.

Figure 1 shows the changes in the levels of infant mortality in the most important social groups, classified by occupational rank, during the period between 1877 and 1914. In order to reduce the effect of the short-term, quasi-cyclical fluctuations in the mortality rates, I have also calculated averages over two and three years. These are shown in Table 4.[45] The period under discussion can be divided into three parts which can be identified most clearly from

45. Groups are defined as follows: self-employed in property, trade or other occupation (including liberal professions up to 1901); public officials (including liberal professions and members of the armed forces from 1902 onwards); private officials and white-collar workers (whose contracts of employment could be terminated); people who regularly sold their labour at hourly or piece rates, mainly journeymen, assistants, apprentices, factory workers (hereafter termed 'skilled workers' for convenience, although, to be accurate, this refers only to a large section of these); people who occasionally sold their labour at hourly or piece rates, mainly day and casual labourers (hereafter termed 'unskilled workers'); people who received wages and payment in kind, i.e. domestics, manservants, maidservants, all other kinds of servant (cf. types of occupation listed in these categories in *Preußische Statistik*, vol. 48 (Berlin, 1879)). Of course, the categories are not entirely clear-cut and it is likely that over time they refer to slightly different groups of people. However, because of the sizes of the groups involved, significant inequalities are bound to be represented.

Figure 1 Infant mortality among various occupational groups in Prussia, 1877–1914 (occupation of father for legitimate, of mother for illegitimate infant)

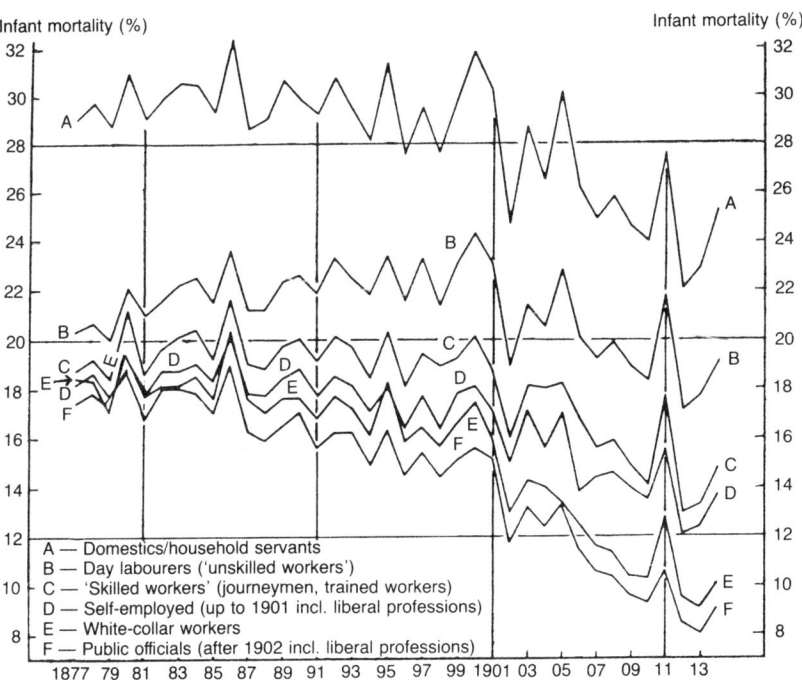

the figures under 'Total population' in Table 4. In the first part, which lasted until about 1886, Germany was still subject to the effects of the take-off of industry, as a result of which the level of infant mortality still tended to be on the increase. In the second part (from 1886 to around 1902) the average infant mortality rates more or less stagnated, while the third and final part (from 1903–6 to 1913) has been described as 'the first period of long-term decline in infant mortality in Germany'.[46]

From an examination of the developmental trends in the various mortality levels (shown most clearly in Figure 1), it is evident that the subdivision of the period under discussion according to the trend in the average infant mortality rate also seems to correspond

---

46. See F. Rott, 'Der Rückgang der Säuglingssterblichkeit' in Grotjahn et al. (eds), *Ergebnisse*, vol. 1, pp. 122–7, who describes typical sets of 'factors of decline' for each period in which mortality rates declined.

to phases in the development of differences between the various social groups. In the first period (i.e. between 1876 and 1886) the mortality rates exhibit similar levels and follow similar courses. In this early phase, social inequality with regard to infant mortality was still relatively low. By 1902–3 the disparities had gradually increased: in Figure 1 the gap widens considerably, reflecting increasing social inequality in the face of death. Although the third period was characterised by a predominantly downward trend, the speed with which the rates fell varied so much that by 1913 the disparities between the various social groups had actually increased further.

The average mortality figures for the years 1877–9 (Table 4) show that the lowest infant mortality rate was in the category of public officials, followed, in ascending order, by the self-employed, white-collar workers, skilled (journeymen and factory workers) or unskilled workers (casual labourers) and, finally, with by far the highest rate, servants and other domestic staff. The fact that the mortality rate for the latter should have been so high was undoubtedly linked to the high proportion of illegitimate children, which fluctuated between 30 and 50 per cent for domestic staff in the country and, as a rule, between 50 and 70 per cent for those in the towns. The conditions that such illegitimate children had to live in were extremely arduous and the mortality rate — especially among infants — was correspondingly high. Leaving this particular group aside for the moment, both because of its relatively untypical life style and because it represented no more than a small percentage of the working population in Prussia, it appears that the levels of infant mortality in the first four social groups actually differed only very slightly.

To emphasise this point I have calculated the infant mortality rates for all of these social groups in seven sample years as a percentage of the mortality rate among infants born to public officials, which remained especially low. Table 5 shows the excess mortality rates. The results show that, in 1877 for example, even among skilled workers excess infant mortality rate was less than 10 per cent. The excess rate among unskilled workers was no more than 17 per cent and was thus only 2 per cent higher than the overall Prussian average. Conversely, the dramatically high rate of infant mortality among servants and domestic staff was already apparent in 1877.

If the differences in the infant mortality rates — which reflect differences in the life chances and in the individual's chances of survival — are any guide, then the advantages enjoyed at the beginning of the period under discussion by public officials (at that time not including the liberal professions) were still very small. These data do not really provide any tangible evidence to suggest that any one group was noticeably privileged in this respect, especially since there was no great difference between the first three social groups and the large group of skilled workers. By the turn of the century, however, the situation had changed considerably. For one thing, a clear disparity had developed between the living conditions of two large sections of the population. In the intervening period, infant mortality levels among public officials, the self-employed and white-collar workers had slightly improved, whereas in all the other categories of workers and domestic staff they had worsened — among unskilled workers by as much as 15 per cent (calculated from the figures in Table 4). Thus, the only groups to have benefited from the modest fall in the infant mortality rates over the first 25 years of the period under discussion were, on average, the self-employed, public officials, white-collar workers and those in the liberal professions. It was not only that the working classes missed out on this improvement: their infants' life chances had actually diminished. The increased disparity was reflected in the corresponding excess mortality rates in the years up to 1900 (see Table 5).

What is even more noticeable, however, is the way in which mortality rates changed during the third part of the period under analysis. Although the rates in all social groups tended to fall in the years after 1903–6, the differences between them actually grew rather than diminished. White-collar workers were the only group that managed to keep within any distance of the public officials as far as their children's life chances were concerned. From the 1890s onwards, the excess mortality rate in this group remained relatively stable at around 11–12 per cent. All other groups saw the disparity between the public officials and themselves grow dramatically. In 1913, the rate for the self-employed amounted to 50 per cent. For skilled workers it was more than 60 per cent, unskilled workers almost 120 per cent and servants and other domestic staff 183 per cent. In the same year the average level of infant mortality in Prussia was 85 per cent higher than the rate among public officials.

Thus, public officials and white-collar workers (including the liberal professions) gained to a disproportionately high degree from the social progress which was reflected in the decline in infant mortality. By 1913, the average rate had fallen by 53 per cent since 1877–9 among public officials, by 50 per cent among white-collar workers, by 32 per cent among the self-employed, by 31 per cent among skilled workers, by 24 per cent among servants and domestic staff and, finally, by 16 per cent among unskilled workers. It is possible therefore to divide society up into three groups, in respect of both the final infant mortality rate and the relative progress made in the long-term reduction of that rate. The first group consists of the public officials, white-collar workers and those in the liberal professions, the second group is made up of the self-employed and skilled workers, and the third of the unskilled workers, servants and other domestic staff.

In view of the fact that these trends became increasingly marked over a 30-year observation period, and affected large sections of the population, it may be concluded that public officials, white-collar workers and the members of the liberal professions (what are termed the 'new middle classes') represented a relatively dynamic social group which was able to improve its market capacity considerably in the last quarter of the nineteenth century. With regard to the indicator we have been using here — i.e. infant mortality — it should be emphasised that this dynamism was likely to have a long-term impact on the distribution of life chances. Furthermore, while in terms of the average for the total Prussian population, skilled workers were certainly in a worse position than public officials, with regard to life chances, which in this case also meant chances of survival, they were clearly distinct from the other section of the working class, unskilled workers. Thus the dividing-line in the social structure separating skilled and unskilled workers seems to have been much more important than that between the various sections of the middle-class and the working-class population as a whole. Although these conclusions are supported by the existing evidence, they are none the less essentially hypothetical in character. This should be emphasised, given their possible implications.[47]

It might be thought — although there are no immediate grounds for so doing — that all that is recorded in a breakdown of the population according to occupational status are differences in wealth and income. However, this view can be countered in the light of the data in Table 6, which reflect the more finely differentiated criteria of occupational status that were used after 1902. The first point worth noting concerns the subdivisions within the

---

47. These theses are firmly supported by the findings of Stearns and Haller et al.: see P.N. Stearns, 'The Unskilled and Industrialization. A Transformation of Consciousness', *Archiv für Sozialgeschichte*, 16 (1976), pp. 250–6; and Haller et al., *Strukturen*, pp. 682, 776–7, and 880–5, which examines the inter-war and post-war periods.

categories of public officials and white-collar workers. For although the lowest infant mortality figures of all were those enjoyed by the senior public officials, who, because most of them had received a university education, could be classed alongside members of the liberal professions, the figures for junior public officials and white-collar workers were comparable and clearly better than the levels for other social groups. The lower levels enjoyed by public officials and white-collar workers cannot therefore simply be explained — and they certainly cannot principally be explained — in terms of differences in wealth, though of course such differences may have produced divisions within these groups. Secondly, I feel it is worth noting that those working in trade and commerce, whether self-employed, blue-collar or white-collar workers, tended to be rather better off than those in manufacturing and craft industries and, more particularly, than those in the agricultural sector. This would seem to confirm the view that the less one's employment was related to agriculture or to a sphere directly concerned with production, the more likely one was to benefit from the social progress which found its expression in improved chances of infant survival. Moreover, a further conclusion that may be drawn from Table 6 is that the difference between infant mortality rates among skilled and unskilled workers was so decisive that the former showed considerable similarity to the self-employed, with skilled workers in trade and commerce in particular proving to be comparable to white-collar workers and junior public officials. In any case, the infant mortality figures among skilled workers in both sectors of the economy were lower than the overall average in both 1902–3 and 1912–13, while those for unskilled workers remained above average throughout the period we are investigating.

In order to be able to identify as precisely as possible the social privileges and deprivations that affected the process of infant care, and which largely determined the level of infant mortality, I distinguished elsewhere between neo-natal and post-natal infant mortality. Whilst the mortality rate within the first month of life (neo-natal) is generally supposed to be more influenced by purely biological determinants, the rate between the second and twelfth months (post-natal), as scholars in the field of social medicine have been emphasising in recent years, is increasingly shaped by exclusively social influences. This view assumes that neo-natal mortality is caused for the most part by premature birth (the infant's inability to live), congenital deformity or defective organs, factors which can hardly be said to have been caused by social deprivation. It is claimed that post-natal mortality, on the other hand, is a function of exposure to infectious diseases and the ability to resist them, and as such appears to be closely linked to the infrastructural and familial environments in which the infant grows up. Even if these arguments merely indicate general trends, it seems safe to assume that the effects of inadequate child care — and thus of the social situation (in the broadest sense of the term) and the life style of the family concerned — are not particularly significant during the infant's first month, but become increasingly dominant during the course of the first year. This assumption is all the more convincing if one remembers that a high percentage of neo-natal deaths occurs during the first few days after birth.

With these considerations in mind, I broke down the infant mortality figures for six administrative districts of the Kingdom of Saxony for the years 1899–1903 according to the social status of the father. In a few selected groups I distinguished between neo-natal and post-natal mortality.[48] It immediately became clear that the average infant mortality rates in Saxony — for the population as a whole and for individual groups — were considerably higher than the corresponding rates in Prussia. Most of them came to some 25–30 per cent, levels which in Prussia at this time (around 1900) were occurring in only the most deprived areas of a few cities, and among very small sections of the population. Even large numbers of public officials and white-collar workers were affected, though of course in the Saxon context they were still relatively fortunate. The differences between the highest and lowest infant mortality rates among public officials and white-collar workers were greater than those in any of the social groups in Prussia. This would indicate that the heterogeneity of the Prussian groups has advantages for analysis, because the statistical weight of the 'leaders' in each group is not so great as to distort the results.

I was also able to calculate the disparities between the levels of infant mortality in the Saxon social groups, taking the rate among public officials as a standard. Distinguishing between neo-natal and post-natal mortality did not alter the fact that this group was more privileged: in both cases their children were the most likely to survive. It is noticeable, however, that when compared to the other social groups, the two working-class categories — skilled and unskilled — were better off with regard to neo-natal mortality than in the case of post-natal death. In respect of the latter, the ranges in the various groups grew in both absolute and relative terms. The

---

48. See Spree, 'Strukturierte soziale Ungleichheit', Tables 9 and 10, pp. 81–2.

point must be taken further, however. It can be shown that the distance separating public officials from the self-employed in agriculture, industry and commerce did not become noticeably greater, whereas that between skilled workers and senior public officials, on the one hand, and between the working-class population as a whole and the self-employed, on the other, certainly did. This seems to confirm the view that the unfavourable living conditions and lower quality of child care in the working-class population did not begin seriously to threaten the child's survival from the first day, but that adverse effects proceeded to make themselves felt during the child's first twelve months. The longer they lived, the greater the disadvantages endured by working-class children became by comparison with their counterparts in other social groups: this may be interpreted as a statistically verifiable process of relative deprivation. In the same way, the advantages enjoyed by the families of senior officials represent relative privilege. My calculations also lead to the conclusion that the favourable living conditions that the children of public officials tended to enjoy were effective from the first day of life, and did not deteriorate to any serious degree during the first 12 months, at least compared to the other social groups. Indeed, the evidence suggests that the opposite occurred: the fact that the proportion of neo-natal deaths in the annual average infant mortality figures was higher among senior public officials than it was in the combined category of skilled and unskilled industrial workers (25 and 23 per cent respectively), is a further indication that the chances a working-class child had of surviving tended to fall in the course of the first 12 months, whereas those of children of public officials increased.

2.4 Infant Mortality and Diet

This section will investigate the various aspects of an indicator which provides more direct information on attitudes to child care: diet. Unfortunately though, there is one fundamental disadvantage with the relevant statistical material on the subject: data on mortality figures are no longer classified according to the criterion of social status. Instead a number of other social criteria come into play, with the result that the discussion cannot be carried on along the same lines as above. In examining diet and methods of nutrition, we are usually interested in the extent or length of time that infants are breast-fed by their mothers. Ever since classical antiquity, there have always been writers who felt that an infant's health was in grave danger if it was fed 'artificially' from an early age — whether with animal milk, gruels or other surrogates — rather than being breast-fed by its mother for as long as possible. There had been continuous debate in Germany since the eighteenth century on the advantages and disadvantages of artificial nutrition (in the broadest sense of the term) by comparison with breast-feeding. All this resulted in a growth in the amount of propaganda in favour of breast-feeding, which by the 1870s and 1880s had reached such levels that it had begun to assume the character of a campaign. Frequent attempts were made to underpin the arguments levelled against all forms of artificial feeding by calling on a mass of statistical data designed to show that infants who had been breast-fed for as long as possible were more likely to survive.[49] After the 1880s, such data tended to be more convincing since from that time onwards the figures on different nutritional methods were actually recorded in terms of mortality rates. Records must also have been made of how surviving infants had been fed. This had not been the case in the preceeding decades, with the result that the corresponding data — that were claimed to refer to mortality figures — did not really represent any reliable rates. More recent studies of the importance of the type of nutrition, and of breast-feeding by the mother in particular, for infants' chances of surviving in developing countries[50] show that the method of nutrition can justifiably be treated as a variable which intervenes in the socio-structural influences on infant mortality that were discussed above.

Leading the way in providing statistical evidence for the link

49. See Duden and Ottmüller, 'Der süße Bronnen'. There are some problems with the way source material is interpreted in U. Ottmüller, 'Speikinder — Gedeihkinder. Kommunikationstheoretische Überlegungen zu Gestalt und Funktion frühkindlicher Sozialisation im bäuerlichen Lebenszusammenhang des deutschsprachigen 19. und frühen 20. Jahrhunderts' (unpubl. diss., Freie Universität Berlin, 1986). For a rather superficial historical account, see A. Ende, 'Zur Geschichte der Stillfeindlichkeit in Deutschland 1850–1978', *Kindheit*, 1 (1979), pp. 203–14. A more general account of infant diets in the nineteenth century is given in H.-J. Teuteberg and A. Bernhard, 'Wandel der Kindernahrung in der Zeit der Industrialisierung' in J. Reulecke and W. Weber (eds), *Fabrik — Familie — Feierabend. Beiträge zur Sozialgeschichte des Alltags* (Wuppertal, 1978), pp. 135–214. From among the extensive contemporary literature, see A. Bluhm, 'Die Stillungsnot, ihre Ursachen und die Vorschläge zu ihrer Bekämpfung. Eine kritische übersicht', *Zeitschrift für soziale Medizin*, 3 (1908); Tugendreich, 'Der Einfluß der sozialen Lage', pp. 270–90. Vincent's statistical evaluation of the literature on breast-feeding in the USA since the end of the nineteenth century is informative, and shows that many countries produced propaganda on breast-feeding: C.E. Vincent, 'Trends in Infant Care Ideas', *Child Development*, 22 (3) (1951), pp. 199–203.

50. Current aspects of the theme, particularly in relation to the developing countries, are discussed in J.E. Knodel and H. Kintner, 'The Impact of Breast Feeding Patterns on the Biometric Analysis of Infant Mortality', *Demography*, 14 (4) (1977). For a similar approach see J.E. Knodel, 'Breast-Feeding and Population Growth', *Science*, 198 (1977), pp. 1111–15.

between diet and infant mortality were the surveys conducted by the Berlin Statistical Office under its director Böckh, who decreed that from 1885 onwards censuses should strive to ascertain how living infants were fed. The results, which were published regularly, make it possible to chart the dangers inherent in artificial feeding over a relatively long period (up to the First World War). From 1885 to 1910 the level of infant mortality amongst Berlin infants fed on substitutes was always many times higher than the rate for breast-fed babies. This trend can be illustrated by taking the figures for two sample years. In 1885 the mortality rate for artificially fed children of married parents was almost seven times higher than the rate for infants who were breast-fed by their mothers. By 1910 this rate had fallen slightly, but was still 4.4 times higher.[51]

Although often imitated, the Böckh method, as it was known, proved to be a considerable strain on administrative resources and was not immune to mistakes or errors. Thus, around the turn of the century, a different approach was adopted in many cases. This involved asking the mothers of all infants born in a sample year and in a particular area (even if they had subsequently died during the course of that year) about the method they used to feed their offspring.[52] As well as being extremely reliable, these surveys had the further advantage that they could be used to ascertain other factors affecting the level of infant mortality in the section of the population under investigation, particularly certain social criteria such as the occupational status and income of the parents, the occupation of the mother, family size and frequency with which the mother had given birth. There is no space here to review such varied information in any depth, but it is possible to summarise the results and give an impression of the overriding patterns that emerge from them.

Table 7 shows how legitimate infants were fed in towns and rural areas in western Germany for the period 1905–11. Groups are classified according to the father's income. At first glance, the results appear confusing. Each income group contains a number of completely different figures for the percentage of infants breast-fed.

---

51. See R. Böckh, 'Tabellen betreffend den Einfluß der Ernährungsweise auf die Kindersterblichkeit', *Bulletin de l'Institut International de Statistique* (1887), vol.2, 2nd edn, pp. 14–24, esp. p. 18; *Statistisches Jahrbuch der Stadt Berlin*, vol. 32 (1908–11), p. 212.

52. For an overview of all surveys of this type carried out before 1912, see Komitee zur Ermittlung der Säuglingsernährung in Hannover-Linden (eds), *Säuglingsernährung, Säuglingssterblichkeit und Säuglingsschutz in den Städten Hannover und Linden* (Berlin, n.d. [1913]), p. 49; see also H. Kintner, 'Trends and Regional Differences in Breast-feeding in Germany from 1871 to 1937', *Journal of Family History*, 27 (2) (1985), pp. 163–82.

To this extent, there are great differences between the various towns and regions under comparison. However, there is a tendency throughout for the level of breast-feeding to fall as income rises. As the averages recorded in columns 10 and 11 show, however, a sharp increase in the level of artificial feeding does not take place until around the 3,000 Mark annual income bracket. Moreover, it is noticeable that in some of the towns and rural districts breast-feeding is very uncommon, even in the lowest income groups. It should not be forgotten that these figures also record extremely short periods of breast-feeding. Consequently, the percentage of breast-fed infants seems to have been exaggerated because, as the original sources indicate, the level of breast-feeding declines sharply in all income groups after the third month.

The significance of breast-feeding for the infant mortality rate can be shown with the help of Tables 8 and 9. It is immediately clear that whatever the income group, the mortality rate increases many times over when breast-feeding is replaced by artificial nutrition. The average increase is 300 per cent in both groups. However, the mortality rate for artificially fed infants in the lower income bracket was as much as 20 percentage points above the corresponding figure in the higher income group. For infants who were artificially fed, the excess mortality rate among children of poorer families was on average 77 per cent. This fell to around 40 per cent if they were breast-fed for at least a few months, though of course this difference is of less social significance in view of the fact that the overall mortality rate is lower in the breast-fed group.

The averages conceal the fact that it is possible to deduce considerable regional variations from the tables. In some cases the excess mortality rate in the lower income group is still much higher even when the infants were breast-fed: in the town of Neuß 110 per cent, in the rural districts of Geldern and Neuß 91 and 88 per cent, and in Hanover 66 per cent. In other cases, on the other hand, the differences between the mortality rates were much smaller as a result of breast-feeding (in Linden the excess rate for the lower income group was 27 per cent, in Rheydt 25 per cent, and in Barmen and Grevenbroich 14 per cent). The general pattern shows therefore that breast-feeding afforded an element of protection against infant mortality: even in the lower-income groups the mortality levels (with the exception of the town of Neuß) fell below 10 per cent. The average infant rates in the Rhenish provinces and the province of Hanover exceeded this level until the early 1920s and in Prussia until the mid-1920s.

There can be no doubt that the lives of infants fed with substitutes were in more danger, especially in the lower-income groups. Such children were more exposed to the unfavourable conditions — and particularly to the risk of infectious disease — that resulted from low income (which makes it impossible to buy high-quality surrogates), poor housing conditions (which make it difficult to ensure that food is stored and meals are prepared in a germ-free environment), and inadequate awareness of the need for nutritional hygiene or for a physiologically balanced diet. One might speak in this context of a poverty syndrome related to the feeding of infants. In the materially and socially more privileged groups, the dangers associated with artificial nutrition must have been correspondingly reduced.

Contrary to modern opinion, and also to the conviction of the medical profession since the 1920s that epidemics, and thus the root of exceedingly high infant mortality, had been successfully eradicated, doctors before the First World War were not at all convinced that medical care or the art of healing in the narrower sense could make any significant contribution to a fall in the overall infant mortality rates — with the exception perhaps of smallpox vaccination. Instead, efforts to reduce infant mortality were guided by the hope that there would be a gradual breakthrough as a result of infrastructural changes introduced to raise the standard of urban hygiene (water supply, sewage disposal, etc.), and that domestic hygiene, social security policies and a system of dispensaries for infants and mothers would improve infants' chances of survival. In particular, much faith was placed in the combination of campaigns encouraging breast-feeding and advice on the ideal forms of substitute nutrition. Since appropriate forms of artificial nutrition tended to be rather expensive, the vast majority of mothers were continually being exhorted to breast-feed their babies by public health officers (during vaccination sessions), by a wide range of charitable organisations (for example at dispensaries for infants and mothers, in leaflets, by peripatetic teachers and press reports, etc.), and by the authorities (for example, when applications were made for maternity benefit, or for supplements paid to women during lactation). In spite of this, the number of breast-fed infants in Berlin, for example, declined rapidly and continuously throughout the period under discussion.[53]

53. See Spree, 'Strukturierte soziale Ungleicheit', Table 14, p. 88. Although Berlin can be regarded as a typical example of a rapidly expanding conurbation with a high proportion of women workers, other places witnessed quite opposite developments. Thus in Munich the incidence of breast-feeding rose from less than 15 per cent in 1880 to over 90 per cent in 1933: see H. Seidlmayer, *Geburtenzahl, Säuglingssterblichkeit und Stillung in München in den letzten 50 Jahren* (Munich, 1937), Tables 14

Apart from the influence of various socio-cultural traditions, the number of mothers who breast-fed their babies was also probably affected by other circumstances such as their occupations, particularly by the specific form their work took and the number of hours they worked. It would be reasonable to assume that the high levels of infant mortality among the working classes and lower-income groups could be interpreted as a consequence of the low incidence of breast-feeding, of the relatively early switch to forms of artificial feeding, and of the higher proportion of working mothers in these groups. Despite the apparent plausibility of this hypothesis, it is very difficult to prove, since I have no statistical material in my possession on the percentage of working women in each group, let alone the proportion of those that were mothers. Similarly, there do not seem to be any infant mortality figures available that have been classified according to how infants were fed, social group and mother's occupation. There are other more general statistics, however, that provide information on how many women breast-fed, and some others that record the reasons given by mothers as to why they decided either not to breast-feed their babies at all or to do so only for a short time. Questions were also asked about the importance of their employment. The information obtained from such inquiries for Barmen, the administrative district of Düsseldorf and for Hanover-Linden is reasonably reliable, and covers the years 1905–12.

One of the first things to emerge is that the percentage of working mothers with legitimate children appears to have been relatively low. The level of employment was never more than 20 per cent, though for unmarried mothers the figure was considerably higher — usually more than 60 per cent. Moreover, it should also be remembered that while these data refer to regular employment which was remunerated, there may in addition well have been other kinds of strenuous labour (such as housework in families with large numbers of children, work in the garden, part-time

---

and 20. On the interaction between doctors and mothers, see, for example, P. Branca, *Silent Sisterhood: Middle Class Women in the Victorian Home* (London, 1975); Ottmüller, ' "Mutterpflichten" '. An account of how smallpox was eradicated as a general cause of death is provided in D.R. Hopkins, *Princes and Peasants. Smallpox in History* (Chicago and London, 1983). For a recent analysis of Germany see J. Brügelmann, 'Medikalisierung von Säuglings- und Erwachsenenalter in Deutschland zu Beginn des 19. Jahrhunderts aufgrund medizinischer Topographien' in A.E. Imhof (ed.), *Leib und Leben in der Geschichte der Neuzeit* (Berlin, 1983), pp. 177–92; idem, 'Der Blick des Arztes auf die Krankheit im Alltag 1779–1850. Medizinische Topographien als Quelle für die Sozialgeschichte des Gesundheitswesens' (unpubl. diss., Freie Universität Berlin, 1982); C. Huerkamp, 'The History of Smallpox Vaccination in Germany: A First Step in the Medicalization of the General Public', *Journal of Contemporary History*, 20 (4) (1985), pp. 617–35.

cleaning jobs and other forms of casual labour) which were not considered to be employment as such, but which none the less made breast-feeding much more difficult. Thus the few available statistics on the subject presumably give a rather distorted picture.

The reasons given by women for stopping breast-feeding present a similar picture. In only 5–15 per cent of cases was work, and taking up employment, given as the reason, an insignificant figure compared with the various physiological factors (such as loss of breast milk for no apparent reason, or sickness of the mother) which accounted for 50–80 per cent of all cases.[54] However, in view of the intensive propaganda campaign in support of breast-feeding and the prevalent social attitudes that were hostile to money-earning mothers, many of them may have felt somewhat reluctant to give the interviewers any other reasons than 'compelling' physiological reasons for their 'failure to fulfil their maternal obligations'. The importance of this particular information should therefore not be exaggerated.

The figures recorded for Hanover-Linden are instructive and relevant. The survey established the numbers of working and non-working mothers who breast-fed their babies, and specified whether work was carried out at home or elsewhere. The most important results are shown in Table 10. These show that even the proportion of legitimate infants who were breast-fed appears to have been very low (around 52 per cent) if the mother was working at home. However this is slightly misleading because the proportion of non-working mothers in Hanover during this period who breast-fed their babies was only 55 per cent. Breast-feeding was markedly less common among mothers who worked outside the home (around 39 per cent). In view of this, the relative number of unmarried mothers who worked at home and breast-fed their offspring was astonishingly high (48 per cent, compared with 49 per cent of unmarried mothers who did not work). The differences become much more pronounced where unmarried mothers worked outside

---

54. See in addition the corresponding figures for 1928 in G. Seiffert, 'Das Nichtstillen in Bayern, seine Ursachen und seine Bekämpfung', *Münchener Medizinische Wochenschrift*, 77 (2) (1930), p. 1198. An impressive analysis of possible socio-economic reasons for why women did not breast-feed, particularly in rural areas, is to be found in W.R. Lee, 'The Impact of Agrarian Change on Women's Work and Child Care in Early Nineteenth-Century Prussia' in J.C. Fout (ed.), *German Women in the Nineteenth Century. A Social History* (New York and London, 1984), pp. 234–55; idem, 'Family and "Modernisation": The Peasant Family and Social Change in Nineteenth-Century Bavaria' in R. Evans and W.R. Lee (eds), *The German Family* (London, 1981), pp. 84–119. Reliable data on women's employment in Germany since the late nineteenth century are also to be found in the recent work by W. Müller et al., *Strukturwandel der Frauenarbeit 1880–1980* (Frankfurt am Main and New York, 1983).

the home. In these cases, only around 20 per cent of infants were being breast-fed.

As is emphasised in note 1 to Table 10, these statistics only applied to a small percentage of all mothers with illegitimate children (the majority had given the children away). They therefore record information relating to mothers who had a particularly strong interest in their children's welfare. However, given that almost half of these mothers worked in factories (compared with 19 per cent of married mothers), and less than 20 per cent of them breast-fed, it would seem that on the whole a relationship exists between breast-feeding and the mother's work environment. The proportion of married mothers in work before the First World War seems to have been so low (in Hanover, for example, they amounted to 15 per cent of the total) that the statistics do not provide evidence to suggest that undertaking paid employment was the reason why mothers did not breast-feed their infants, or weaned their children at a very early age. Since, moreover, about half of all such work was done at home, there were opportunities to continue breast-feeding. On the other hand, the very small numbers of women who worked in factories or elsewhere outside the home and who breast-fed their babies makes it clear that this type of regular employment was a serious obstacle to breast-feeding. Thus, if a woman worked in a factory, the chances of her being able to breast-feed her baby were slim. This was also reflected in the demands made at the time for the provision of rooms at the workplace where women could breast-feed their babies. Such facilities remained extremely rare before the First World War, and anyhow were of little use in themselves without the simultaneous provision of a crèche. In relation to the total number of mothers, however, only a few were concerned with such issues, so this cannot be cited as an explanation of the differences between the levels of infant mortality specific to each social group.

Another approach consists of testing whether breast-feeding was less common or terminated at an earlier stage in the working-class population than elsewhere. The figures from Table 7 show that more working-class women tended to breast-feed their babies than women from other social groups — at least during the first few months. The overwhelming majority of people in the income group with the highest level of breast-feeding (i.e. under 1500 Marks per year) were working-class. More specific information was recorded in the town of Barmen (in 1905), in which occupational status and income were combined. These figures reveal that 54 per cent of the fathers of children under the age of 12 months from the group of public officials and the liberal professions had an income of less than 1500 Marks. Fifty-nine per cent of all white-collar workers, 61 per cent of the self-employed and 100 per cent of all categories of blue-collar worker also fell into this income bracket.[55] Conversely, 82 per cent of working-class infants were breast-fed, the highest proportion of all groups. This figure should not, however, be regarded as the norm for working-class women everywhere: the average calculated for a whole series of cities and rural districts in western Germany indicates that no more than around two-thirds of working-class women breast-fed during the first few months (cf. Table 7). In Mönchengladbach this figure was little more than 50 per cent, which shows that there was considerable regional variation. On the basis of these surveys, the only possible conclusion, as I see it, that can be reached — and this means going beyond the information reproduced in Table 7 — is that there is little substantial evidence to prove that working-class children were more likely to die during their first 12 months than children from other social groups because they were not breast-fed. (Illegitimate children were excluded from our calculations because, as we indicated above, the situation in their case was different.)

One possibility might have been, however, that working-class children were weaned too early. Unfortunately, the information contained in existing empirical studies on this subject is inadequate. The rather more extensive material that has been processed in Table 11 records the percentages of legitimate infants that were breast-fed and the duration of breast-feeding, divided into two groups according to the father's income. Since the figures emphasise regional variations, it would appear more sensible to analyse the figures for one particular region. The pattern that emerges is none the less unambiguous: up to the end of the third month the incidence of breast-feeding was approximately the same in both income groups, but from then on the differences between them became more marked. As a rule, the infants from the higher-income group tended to be weaned earlier than those from the lower group, though there does not seem to have been any reason for this other than convention. This trend varied in strength from region to region: it was most marked in Barmen and weakest in Hanover-Linden. Assuming that the overwhelming majority of fathers with an annual net income of less than 1500 Marks (or in Hanover less than 1800 Marks) were workers, it may be tentatively concluded

---

55. See Kriege und Seutemann, 'Ernährungsverhältnisse und Sterblichkeit der Säuglinge in Barmen', *Centralblatt für allgemeine Gesundheitspflege, 25* (1906), p. 22.

that it is impossible to judge whether or not the infants of working-class parents (in view of their poor-quality housing and low standard of living, and the difficulties they experienced in guaranteeing a quantitively and hygienically ideal form of artificial nutrition) were weaned too early. Moreover, there are no convincing grounds for assuming that working-class women tended to breast-feed their infants less or wean them earlier than women from other social groups. On the contrary, there is good reason to believe that working-class infants were more likely to be fed with their mothers' milk and for a longer period than infants from other social groups.

These conclusions are substantiated by the figures in Table 12, which directly compares the average levels and duration of breast-feeding prevalent in each group (in Hanover-Linden in 1912). The slight changes in the picture from the image projected hitherto are not without interest. For although working-class women in Hanover-Linden were much slower in weaning their infants after the third month than the wives of the self-employed or academics, until as late as the ninth month breast-feeding was as common among wives of middle-level and junior officials as it was among working-class women — and indeed it was sometimes even more common. In this respect, then, middle-class women tended to follow the example of working-class mothers in their breast-feeding habits rather than the social model provided by the wives of senior public officials.

2.5 Recapitulation

I shall now summarise the evidence concerning the significance of diet and methods of nutrition as intervening variables affecting infant mortality. The initial overriding impression was that the level of infant mortality was inversely proportional to the level of wealth: the greater the wealth, the lower the mortality rate, and vice versa. Assuming wealth to be an approximate indicator of market capacity, then this relation would have to be interpreted as a reflection of the fact that the differences between the various infant mortality rates depended directly on class differences. If this were true, varying infant mortality rates would be no more than signs of different class positions. By taking methods of nutrition into consideration, however, I was able to show that it is not only theoretically unconvincing, but also statistically untenable, to assume that there is a direct relationship between wealth and mortality, and thus between class position and infant mortality. Breast-feeding an infant for as long as possible during its first 12 months provided excellent protection against infection (we should recall that the main causes of death among infants before the First World War were infections of the stomach and intestines). If the mother was engaged in some form of employment, especially outside the home, then she found it much more difficult to breast-feed — particularly in the case of factory-work. Before the First World War, however, the number of married women to whom this applied was still relatively low. Consequently, the statistical significance of any rise in infant mortality that may have occurred because married mothers worked outside the home is virtually negligible. On the other hand, the other factors that may have prevented mothers from breast-feeding their babies, particularly in the lower-income groups, have not been thoroughly enough researched for us to be able to propose any more conclusive hypotheses. Although we have rejected the idea that infant mortality was determined directly by class, this does not preclude the possibility that there may have been a number of more indirect links which it might be possible to clarify in future analyses.

For the moment, though, there is one rather obvious conclusion: individual variables such as income, size of living space, the standard of domestic hygiene and level of education, and so on, can be used only in a limited way to explain differences in mortality rates among the various social groups we have been examining. There is undoubtedly a certain degree of interdependence between these variables, particularly if they are viewed as what Max Weber terms the 'causal components of the market situation'. It might be appropriate to refer to a poverty syndrome: to the accumulation of all the undesirable outcomes of the factors which determine mortality in the lower social groups. What might be obscured by this sort of approach are the small, but socially perhaps most significant nuances which recur repeatedly in the statistical data. These are, for example: the sharp fall in the infant mortality rates even among middle-level and junior public officials and white-collar workers after the turn of the century — in other words, as far as infant mortality was concerned, the poverty syndrome did not affect the expanding 'new middle classes', the majority of whom had limited economic means; the large disparity in infant mortality rates between skilled and unskilled workers, which was considerably larger than the gap separating skilled workers and the middle classes; and the tendency of middle-class mothers with a small housekeeping budget to breast-feed their babies to a degree and for an average length of time that was more 'typical' of working-class behaviour.

This is not to deny the fact that working-class children had fewer life chances and were less likely to survive. It is not difficult to paint a picture of overall *relative* deprivation. However, as long as the relative position of a particular group in the social distribution of privilege or deprivation remains constant, the social scientist who adopts this approach runs the risk of overlooking evidence of concrete changes in the life conditions typical of that group. Placing emphasis on the privilege syndrome, on the one hand, and the poverty syndrome on the other — that is on the great discrepancies between the life chances of various social groups — may prompt the conclusion that inequalities rooted in the social structure can be only resolved by profound social transformation, which the large class organisations or mass movements alone can consciously engineer. As a result, there are bound to be political ramifications if social science takes the view that structures of social inequality have remained remarkably durable for a long period of time.[56] For this reason it should be stated all the more strongly that overemphasising the relative position of specific social groups in the social structure can lead to distorted conclusions. Expressed in more political terms, the effect of such overemphasis is to underestimate or dismiss as unimportant the unorganised efforts made by individuals and small groups to improve their positions in certain areas of their lives, particularly in the sphere of private reproduction and with regard to the way children are brought up and educated. The problem is that the efforts of individuals are regarded as rather fragmentary, and thus incapable of exerting a real influence on the structure of social inequality.

If one disregards cases of individual social advancement, it may be quite correct not to expect changes in reproductive behaviour to set a process of levelling in motion, or to cause relative social positions to be reversed, even if the behaviour of large groups is involved. However, it would be erroneous to deny how important

---

56. In this sense see, for example, the resumé of a study of the relationship between social mobility and educational behaviour in Austria over the past 50 years: M. Haller, *Egalisierung der Chancen oder Statusreproduktion? Bildungsexpansion und die Entwicklung der Strukturen sozialer Ungleichheit in Österreich 1933–1972* (Institut für Höhere Studien, Forschungsbericht no. 144 (Vienna, 1979), pp. 84, 100, 109–10. For a similar approach see Handl et al., *Klassenlagen*, pp. 100 and 231–2. In my opinion there is a methodological problem here. These investigations, while constantly stressing the relative positions of individuals and groups in the matrix of social inequality, tend to neglect improvements in absolute levels affecting all groups (although to different degrees), even though it may be the case that potentially such improvements can lead to long-term changes in structures of inequality. This is tentatively broached by Haller, *Egalisierung*, p. 112.

concrete changes in the values, social orientations and patterns of behaviour evidenced in reproduction can be for the perception of social inequality, for the articulation of interests and demands, or for political organisation — in short, for conceptions of the forms and substance of social conflict.

It can be presumed that during the course of the period we are examining, there were considerable improvements in the basic social environment of the lower social strata and in their children's chances of surviving — in other words, in their market capacity or position — precisely because reproductive behaviour was subjected to more rational control and became more deliberate. The lower classes had generally been associated with an allegedly naïve pattern of reproductive behaviour which largely dispensed with conscious birth control and family planning, and with fatalistic acceptance of extreme poverty and large numbers of children. The departure from this pattern of behaviour, together with the more expedient use of the normally extremely modest domestic budget, probably increased, if only by a small amount, the time and financial resources available to each member of the family. Consequently, the chances of children from the lower strata surviving to adulthood also improved. In more general terms, even though new attitudes began to take root only after between one and one and a half generations, people began to have new expectations of what their lives would bring: they became orientated towards a planned future,[57] which rendered it possible and sensible to make 'investments' in children (for example in the form of a longer and better education).

There is absolutely no doubt that by the 1920s the German working class had begun to rationalise its private life in this way, and that since the 1950s this process has continued at a higher level and more rapidly. What is open to question, however, is whether the 'new middle classes' led the way or even assumed an exemplary position in this respect during the last years of the Wilhelmine Empire, and to what extent similar patterns could already be perceived in the working class. The existence of such parallels in the psychological and behavioural changes and reorientations in various social groups cannot be taken for granted. Rises in real incomes above certain thresholds and the stabilisation of both

---

57. For a detailed and balanced view, see J. Müller, 'Geburtenrückgang' in *Handwörterbuch der Staatswissenschaften* (Jena, 1927), 4th edn, vol. 4, pp. 641–7. See also A. v. Nell, 'Die Entwicklung der generativen Strukturen bürgerlicher und bäuerlicher Familien von 1750 bis zur Gegenwart' (unpubl. diss., Bochum, 1973), pp. 11–18, and the literature cited.

wages and the supply of material goods are probably influential factors in the emergence of more rational attitudes and more long-term planning. However, it is open to question whether these thresholds had been reached by the First World War, at least by sections of the working class.

I do not intend to pursue these questions in depth or with the degree of sophistication which would be necessary to reach firm conclusions. Instead, I shall conclude with some additional data on different family sizes — a further intervening variable affecting the mortality rate — which serve to throw some light on the problems I have outlined.

2.6 Infant Mortality and Birth Control

In accordance with the discussion so far, I am assuming that an indirect relationship exists between the average number of children per marriage and the infant mortality rate, and that this relationship is mediated by a number of complex mechanisms. I would now like to provide evidence which will help to illustrate this. I hope that I will be able to clarify this assumption further by examining the major demographic trend of the period we are dealing with: the gradual fall in the birth-rate, which Germany experienced from the 1870s onwards. Although, for the period up until the 1890s, the fall may be interpreted as part of a long-term cycle, I am particularly interested in examining how it varied among different social strata. Although, admittedly, much has been written about such variations, the statistical evidence provided has tended on the whole to be unsatisfactory.

An exception to this rule is the work of Adelheid von Nell (now Gräfin zu Castell), based on the genealogies of families in Lower Saxony. The material she uses is not only relatively wide-ranging but, more importantly, covers a long time-span.[58] Table 13 shows

---

58. See von Nell, 'Die Entwicklung', esp. pp. 141–2; M. Stürzbecher, 'Die Bekämpfung des Geburtenrückganges und der Säuglingssterblichkeit im Spiegel der Reichstagsdebatten 1900–1930. Ein Beitrag zur Geschichte der Bevölkerungspolitik' (unpubl. diss. Freie Universität Berlin, 1954), pp. 3–12. By examining indicators of fertility, Knodel's conclusion is that between 1888–92 and 1931–5 rates declined as follows: overall birth rate by 55 per cent, overall fertility rate by 59 per cent (standardised, as are all of Knodel's indices of fertility, to the fertility rate of the Hutterites), legitimate fertility by 63 per cent and illegitimate fertility by 53 per cent: see Knodel, *The Decline of Fertility*, p. 39. For a critique of these see G. Hohorst, 'The Decline of Fertility Once Again: A Critical Note on John Knodel's Book and Standardized Demographic Indexes', *Historical Social Research — Quantum Information*, 22 (1982), pp. 50–62. During this period the overall number of marriages rose by 18 per cent, while the age at which women first married dropped slightly. See

some of her main conclusions that are of relevance for our purposes. Three large social groups are distinguished within the bourgeois and agricultural middle strata: land-owning farmers, the self-employed in trade and commerce, and the 'new middle classes' (consisting of public officials, officers in the armed forces, the liberal professions, and white-collar workers). Emphasis must be laid on the fact that, as far as the evidence shows, family sizes within these middle-class groups had begun to decline from as early as the beginning of the nineteenth century. Even before industrialisation began to take off, the average number of children had already fallen from between five and six to between four and five in the families of public officials, army officers and academics in the liberal professions (referred to below as 'the educated classes') and the self-employed. The figures for landowning farmers fell from between six and seven to between five and six. By the turn of the century, families of the 'new middle classes' and the self-employed had an average of less than three children, and those of farmers between three and four. Thus, during the nineteenth century the average number of children born to these groups had on the whole fallen by half.

A number of different methods were used to record and classify the statistical data which we will examine in some detail below.[59] The figures shown in Tables 14–17 can be regarded as representative for Germany since they are taken from a survey conducted in 1939 and covering the entire population of the German Reich. One of the drawbacks is that the data essentially refer only to the period beginning in the late 1890s. However, in order to lend more emphasis to the apparent trends in patterns of reproductive behaviour in the decades preceding the First World War, figures for the war years and after have been included despite the fact that, strictly speaking, they do not really belong to the period under analysis.

W.R. Lee, 'Germany' in Lee (ed.), *European Demography and Economic Growth* (London, 1979), pp. 164ff; P. Marschalck, *Bevölkerungsgeschichte Deutschlands im 19. und 20. Jahrhundert* (Frankfurt am Main, 1984), particularly pp. 122–7.

59. *Volkszählung. Die Familien im Deutschen Reich*, compiled by the Statistisches Reichsamt (Berlin, 1943) (= 'Volks-, Berufs- und Betriebszählung von 17.5.1939', *Statistik des Deutschen Reichs*, vol. 554). Survey includes Austria. Data on the number of children per marriage were collected retrospectively in this census. Respondents were asked to indicate how many children each marriage had produced. In the analysis which follows, trends within each cohort will be regarded as effects of the period of time. This is justified if one considers that in most cases, even before 1900, 66–75 per cent of all children were born in the first ten years of the marriage. After 1918, the figure was around 90 per cent. Thus it can be assumed that the couples who married between 1925 and 1929 had already completed their reproductive phase by the time the census was conducted in 1939. Cf. also the statistics in Spree, 'The German Petite Bourgeoisie', pp. 17 and 24–5.

The tables give information on cohorts by year of marriage.

Table 14 provides an initial and approximate picture of social differences. A comparison between the agricultural and urban populations, subdivided into various occupational categories, shows that from the late nineteenth century onwards the fall in the birth rate had been affecting all occupational groups in the agricultural population. However, in each cohort, the number of children was higher in the rural than in the urban population. Rural families had almost one child more than urban families at the beginning of the period (among those who had married before 1905), with the ratio growing from 121:100 to 151:100 (compared with the marriage cohort 1920–4).

Though the birth rate did decline in the rural population, it did so at a slower rate. Consequently, up to the 1920s, differences in fertility between the rural and urban populations grew. On the whole, it is evident that from the late 1920s the average numbers of children born to parents in each occupational group tended to even out throughout the population.

A further question concerns the effect of the size of the community. The calculation in Table 15 shows that in fact the larger the community, the smaller the number of children born to members of each occupational group tended to be. It is interesting to note that discrepancies between the average numbers of children born to public officials and white-collar workers were visible in larger communities. In smaller communities, however, these groups had equal numbers of children. Furthermore, in cities with at least 200,000 inhabitants, blue-collar workers and the self-employed, groups which on the whole produced more children, tended to have fewer children than white-collar workers and public officials from small and medium-sized communities. If community size can be regarded as an indicator of different forms of existence, working conditions and social orientations, then the considerable disparities in the numbers of children produced within each group would suggest that blue-collar workers and the self-employed reacted most strongly to their environments.

Thus far we have been speaking on a very general level, using aggregate figures. Below, these statements will be differentiated on the basis of statistics for 64 occupational groups. The tables show data for 43 of these. Consequently, it is possible to analyse in some detail the role that social differences played in the fall in the birth rate in late nineteenth- and early twentieth-century Germany, and how these differences changed over time. From this point on, however, we do not possess figures which enable us to differentiate between town and country or in terms of community size. Table 16 provides an overview of the survey of families in the Reich. What is apparent is that in all 43 occupational groups there was a consistent fall throughout the period in the number of children per marriage. It is important to mention some of the characteristics of the first cohort — those who married before 1905 — since they represent the initial state of affairs in the pattern of falling fertility.

— By the turn of the century, rural workers were the only group still producing six or more children on average.
— Four groups had between five and six: independent farmers, miners, workers in the stone, glass and ceramics industries, and skilled and unskilled construction workers.
— In 13 occupations, the figure was between four and five (this was also the overall average). These included the self-employed in the 'old middle classes' (excluding traders), all other categories of worker (excluding those in the printing industry), and one group of German public officials: train drivers and guards.
— In the first cohort, public officials (excluding train drivers, etc.), white-collar workers and those in the liberal professions produced the fewest children. The average figure was between two and four, and thus below the mean for the population.
— None of the groups in this cohort produced on average less than two children.

The general picture is a familiar one. There were particularly few children in the families of public officials, white-collar workers and those in the liberal professions. This was also generally true for academics. In contrast, agricultural and blue-collar workers had many children. However, the picture also shows quite considerable differences in the levels of fertility both within and between the major occupational groups. In the first cohort the maximum difference was four children (between agricultural workers and army officers, who had the least children). The vast majority of blue-collar workers had on average about two children more than public officials and white-collar workers.

It is important to establish whether these differences persisted after the First World War. In terms of the absolute numbers of children produced, the answer is clearly that they did not. From the early 1920s onwards, the range in the average numbers of children was distinctly narrower than in the pre-war period. In all occupational groups the numbers lay between one and less than three, the largest difference between them being 1.9. However, relative differences did grow. Comparing the first cohort with the last, the range had risen from 83 per cent to 95 per cent. A further question we might ask is whether the birth-rates in the groups continued to fall in the same sequence. We can use Table 16 to establish who in each cohort produced the least and the most children. Comparing the last and the first cohorts, it appears that almost all the groups which originally produced the fewest (in this case the average was 2.8 or less) had changed by 1925–9 (here the upper limit was 1.6). Whereas, in the first cohort, academics and other self-employed professionals were the least fertile, this was not at all so in the 1925–9 cohort (with the exception of freelance writers and artists, army officers and apothecaries). At the turn of the century, the other end of the range was occupied almost without exception by blue-collar workers and the agricultural population. The 1920–4 cohort, however, represents the final stage of a pattern which had begun to develop before the First World War. Since then, the fewest children have tended to be found among white-collar workers and public officials with medium and low levels of qualifications, certain professionals (on the whole non-academics), some of the self-employed, particularly in trade, and some, particularly skilled and usually urban, blue-collar workers. In contrast, birth-rates among academics and senior public officials declined at a slower rate, with the result that from the 1920s onwards the numbers of children they were producing was similar to the overall average.

The figures in Table 17 show the distribution of married couples in each of the 43 occupational groups with respect to the numbers of children they produced. The percentages allow us to arrive at indicators of the frequency of various family sizes and thus of what can be considered a normative pattern in each case. An examination of the first cohort reveals the following:

— There were considerable differences between groups in terms of the frequency of very large or very small families (including those with no children).
— In the first cohort, there was a 24 percentage-point difference among occupational groups (between 4 and 28 per cent) in the frequency of marriages which bore no children. Childless marriages were particularly frequent among senior and junior army officers, self-employed doctors, writers and artists, university lecturers and judges in the civil service, and so on. Among non-academic white-collar workers and blue-collar workers in the printing industry, the figure was not quite so high, but still above the national average.

- There were also comparable differences between occupational groups in respect of the relative numbers of families with one and two children. On the whole, groups with a high proportion of childless couples also had many with one or two children.
- The proportion of three- and four-child families was relatively similar in all occupational groups.
- After five and more children, the differences widened rapidly.
- There were extreme differences between groups with regard to very large families. These are not included in Table 17. In certain occupations around the turn of the century, more than 10 per cent of families consisted of ten and more children (agricultural workers 17 per cent, independent farmers 14 per cent, miners 14 per cent, workers in the stone, glass and ceramics industries 12 per cent, construction workers 12 per cent). However, in the groups which may be regarded as the harbingers of the decline in the birth-rate, only 4 per cent of families were as large as this.
- Apart from a few exceptions, there are signs in the first cohort that the distribution of 'family size models' among status groups followed a pyramidal shape.

A closer look at Table 17 shows that over the period we are concerned with some shifts occurred in the distribution of 'family size models'. Firstly, the percentage of families with at least ten children declined very sharply. However, in the groups which had previously tended to produce large families, people continued to have at least five children, and thus remained above the average. Considerable differences arose in the proportions of childless couples: there were relatively few in groups which generally had larger families, but in the harbingers of birth-rate decline, the number of these couples continued to rise. There is evidence, however, that the whole population was growing similar in this respect. If we look at the percentage of families with between two and four children, the gaps between the various groups were clearly becoming narrower. The gap was at its narrowest in the case of two children. With the overall percentage rising from 13 to 25 per cent, families of this size were becoming much more common throughout the population.

Let us take a brief look at the different speeds at which the small family became society's established norm.

- In all occupational groups, there were relatively few couples

who had married before the First World War and had not more than one child. Most had three or four.
— During the war and in the years immediately following, the two-child family became the norm amongst independent academics, senior and middle-level white-collar workers, and blue-collar workers in the printing industry. (The criterion is that 75 per cent of all married couples in the group had no more than two children.) Even before 1914 this had been the most common family size in these groups (more than 50 per cent).
— By the end of the 1920s, after a lag of some five to ten years, two children also became the norm for the self-employed in trade and commerce, most middle-level and junior public officials, junior white-collar workers and foremen.
— By contrast, three or more children remained the norm until well into the 1930s among all those working in agriculture, the rest of the self-employed in trade, all blue-collar workers (except those in the printing industry), some groups of academic public officials (church officials, doctors, university lecturers and primary and secondary school teachers), and train drivers and guards.

What can be established with certainty is that after the First World War, the harbinger groups, who in the nineteenth century had led the fall in the birth-rate, were divided when the norm became two or fewer children. Some of the erstwhile trend-setters adhered to a norm that other groups, which can be regarded as late-comers, were exceeding in some instances before, but in any case after, the War. These groups, which from the 1920s onwards were slowing down the fall in the birth-rate, came, on the one hand, from the upper third of the status and income hierarchy, and, on the other, from the lower third. In other words, before the Second World War, the distribution of families who regarded more than two children as the norm began to assume the U-shaped pattern similar to that in evidence over the last few decades. Since 1914, the families in Germany with the least children have come from the middle and lower-middle class, strata which have grown steadily in relation to the rest of the population.

Having discussed the fall in the birth-rate which, though in evidence throughout society, varied across social groups, we should now attempt to establish whether it was connected with infant and child mortality. The hypothesis that parents limited their fertility as a psychological response to their children growing up, postulates that there is in fact a connection here. Indeed for some students of

Changes in Health and Mortality

the subject, it explains the decline in the birth-rate. In its simplest form the theory holds that as long as the relative numbers of children who reach the age of five, or even ten, do not tangibly increase, a long-term decline in fertility cannot generally be expected.[60] Infant and child mortality rates have to fall for a period of between a half and a whole generation before having any effect on fertility. In Knodel's view, it is impossible either to confirm or refute this hypothesis with any certainty on the basis of aggregate figures. He comes to the conclusion that, while in the German Reich as a whole and in most administrative regions the birth-rate and infant mortality rate both fell at the same time, there are no grounds for saying that the one rate influenced the other. However, almost 40 per cent of the overall decline in fertility in the Reich was compensated by lower infant mortality. The detailed calculations made by Meerwarth on the rate of surviving children in relation to births also confirm the thesis that mortality and fertility rates followed each other, but once again do not point to the dominance of either.[61]

I have made some calculations for Prussia, but unlike Knodel I have investigated the differences between social groups rather than regions. Taking Prussia as a whole, it is evident that during the latter part of the nineteenth century fewer children were dying at an early age. This may have sparked off the fall in the birth-rate, or at least contributed to it. On the other hand, the data suggest that even around 1880, the children who were most likely to survive up to the age of five or ten years were in what have been termed the harbinger groups leading the decline in fertility. In fact by the end of the century the advantages they had over children from other social groups had grown even further. Thus a picture of increasing social inequality can be gained by looking not only at infant mortality rates, but also at the chances young children had of surviving. The fact that workers had the least opportunity of improving their children's chances of survival could be cited as a

---

60. A rigid interpretation of the survival hypothesis is found in H. Linde, 'Familie und Haushalt als Gegenstand bevölkerungsgeschichtlicher Forschung. Erörterung eines problembezogenen und materialorientierten Bezugsrahmens' in W. Conze (ed.), *Sozialgeschichte der Familie in der Neuzeit Europas. Neue Forschungen* (Stuttgart, 1976), p. 40. For a general discussion on the determinants of fertility see A.J. Coale and S.C. Watkins (eds), *The Decline of Fertility in Europe* (Princeton and New York, 1986); C. Höhn et al. (eds), *Determinants of Fertility Trends. Theories Reexamined*, (Liège, 1982); S. Preston (ed.), *The Effects of Infant and Child Mortality on Fertility* (New York, 1977).

61. See Knodel, *The Decline of Fertility*, pp. 185ff; R. Meerwarth, 'Die Entwicklung der Bevölkerung während der Kriegs- und Nachkriegszeit' in Meerwarth et al., *Die Einwirkungen des Krieges auf Bevölkerungsbewegung, Einkommen und Lebenshaltung in Deutschland* (Stuttgart, 1932), pp. 22–3.

reason why their fertility declined later than other groups. However, since my material only dates back to about 1880, even an examination of the decline in fertility on a socially differentiated basis is not adequate for testing whether infant mortality rates dominated fertility or vice versa.

On the basis of his recent investigations, Knodel argues that the hypothesis has to be interpreted in a radically individual sense. He recently published a study of the demographic transition in a sample of 14 villages in various parts of Germany from 1750 to 1900.[62] By reconstructing families using village records, he arrives at several main conclusions:

(1) Since the course of demographic transition varies so greatly from village to village, there seems to be little sense in speaking of averages. Knodel suggests it is preferable to speak of a number of 'demographic transitions'.

(2) The fertility levels in many villages had risen by the end of the century; Knodel ascribes this to greater fecundity.

(3) The 'modernisation' of reproductive behaviour — the adoption of birth control — did not take the form of spacing, but of more determined efforts not to have more than a certain number of children (parity-dependent control). This is reflected in the lower ages at which married women bore their last child.

(4) Variations in changes in fertility and in the 'modernisation' of reproductive behaviour were smaller between occupational groups than between regions. It was not until 1850–1900 that such social differences began to make themselves felt — in other words at a time when birth control was becoming generally more common. Fertility varied little with occupation, although the degree to which birth control was practised varied more closely. In general terms it seems, for example, that peasants used birth control most, followed by artisans and the self-employed, with rural workers the least likely to do so.

(5) In his work of 1974 on the decline of fertility in Germany, Knodel rejected the hypothesis that fertility is determined by a proceeding decline in infant mortality as an implausible explanation of the falling birth-rate. After his study of villages, his current position is that some evidence for a variant of the hypothesis can be

62. See J. Knodel, 'Demographic Transitions in German Villages' in Coale and Watkins, *The Decline of Fertility*; idem., 'Child Mortality and Reproductive Behaviour in German Village Populations in the Past: A Micro-Level Analysis of the Replacement Effect', *Population Studies*, 36(2) (1982), pp. 199–200; idem. and C. Wilson, 'The Secular Increase in Fecundity in German Village Populations: An Analysis of Reproductive Histories of Couples Married 1750–1899', *Population Studies*, 35(1) (1981), pp. 68 and 73ff.

found, if it is regarded as applying to individual couples. At this level, the assumption is that those couples whose offspring were surviving were the first to begin to practise birth control. In doing so, they were reacting only to the greater chances *their* children had of surviving — which was most relevant to them — even if the mortality rate of children in their environment (in the village, and more especially in the larger region) remained high.

There are in my opinion a number of weaknesses in the hypothesis we have been discussing, which are not really removed by Knodel's attempt to 'individualise' it:

(1) It ignores the considerable differences in the average numbers of children in occupational or social groups which existed before the overall decline in the birth-rate set in. If such differences are to be regarded as evidence of norms of average family sizes which vary because of social factors, then the question which must be asked is how these norms were related to expectations about how long children would survive, and why in the long term the norms for the different groups grew closer together.

(2) The hypothesis does not provide a satisfactory explanation of why fertility declined in the first half of the nineteenth century. Since this was a period during which the great mass of the population was impoverished, it is highly unlikely that there was an increase in the chances that infants and young children in the population as a whole had of surviving.

(3) The same argument applies to the decline in fertility that occurred at an early stage among public officials and those in the liberal professions. Adelheid von Nell was able to show convincingly that even from the beginning of the nineteenth century the birth-rate among these groups was steadily falling (see Table 13). This is to be seen in connection with the fact that a modern, professional civil service was being established, and certain educated, middle-class groups were consolidating their social position by adopting a rationalistic life style. They valued investment in human capital (especially education) and therefore limited the size of their families.

In opposition to the hypothesis discussed above, I wish to emphasise the significance for reproductive behaviour of changes in the concrete and tangible circumstances of people's lives and occupations. Recently Haines provided firm evidence of the factors which are important here, and elaborated a model.[63] It suffices for

---

63. See M. Haines, *Fertility and Occupation. Population Patterns in Industrialization* (New York, 1979), pp. 37–57.

our purposes to list the main features of the model: origin (above all economic, i.e. whether from the agricultural or the non-agricultural sector); expected income (level and distribution over lifespan); chances of employment (labour market for men); chances for women on the labour market; ratio of the sexes among people of marrying age (marriage market); frequency of child labour; differences in morbidity and mortality, if possible by age; residential structures (economic components such as small-scale farming, access to gardens); and cultural and social components such as the shape of the neighbourhood and circles of relatives. It seems to me that the common link between these factors and fertility is one of *mentality types*. By this term, I understand patterns of attitudes and values which correlate with a particular life style, and which affect reproductive behaviour.

My main objections are directed principally against the 'strong' assumption that the decisive cause of the fall in the birth-rate is the changes in parental experiences of a growing number of children surviving. The contention here, on the other hand, is that fertility may decline even if the chances of offspring surviving do not alter — in other words, even if high infant and child mortality rates persist. I hold that, at the very least, the reduction in fertility is to a great extent independent of these factors, and I believe this to be so, because it is in fact based on changes in mentality.[64] I do not intend to propose this as a hypothesis which excludes all other approaches, by regarding such mentalities as part of the factors listed by Haines. My point is rather that mentalities can influence the development of fertility such that to a certain degree it becomes independent of infant mortality.

By way of example, I believe that examining changes in mentalities provides the key to linking the diverse occupational groups which comprised the harbingers of the decline in fertility. They were academics, artists, senior and middle-level white-collar workers in commerce, the self-employed in trade, and workers and auxiliary workers in the printing industry. There is no doubt that these groups cannot be said to form a social stratum in the traditional sense of the term. They do not have the same social status, nor can they be expected to have earned comparable incomes. But it would seem that the similarities in their reproductive behaviour — at least with regard to the rate and timing of the decline in fertility — can be traced back to their lives and working environments typically sharing certain common, mentality-forming

---

64. On this see also Imhof, *Die gewonnenen Jahre*, pp. 62–73.

characteristics. Above all, these are typically urban occupations which in comparison with others of similar status demand particularly long periods of training and qualification. On the whole, work in these areas involves exercising control over people and things, either in the form of actual control, or by way of language and other symbolic media. In themselves, the occupations are relatively unspecific, and the people in them to a fairly large extent possess qualifications that are not related to their specific work functions, such as adaptability and mobility. In addition, they identify strongly with the ideology of achievement fundamental to industrial societies, and their behaviour both at work and in private expresses an overriding tendency to instrumental rationality. Finally, these are tertiary occupations (even if they are carried out in other sectors of the economy). Thus they are far removed from agriculture, first-hand experience of nature, and spheres of direct production.

Of course, this discussion must be seen as a series of speculative attempts to point out some conditions of life and work which affected the mentalities of social groups exposed to them, and which thus may have given rise to similar patterns of reproductive behaviour. It is particularly important to establish in some detail why it was that under the conditions of nineteenth-century society, rationalist mentalities of this type may have caused the birth-rate to fall. There is, however, no space here to go into that.[65] None the less, there are grounds for concluding that my findings also allow for the possibility that some people reacted to their environments in ways which do not fit in with the general pattern. Thus from the late 1920s onwards, some groups of graduate public officials and a large section of the self-employed in trade showed signs of resisting the continued decline in fertility, and of adhering to a norm of two or three children. It is an example of a variation of the rationalist mentality type, and one which links together heterogeneous occupational groups.

2.7 Hypotheses on the Interrelation between Market Capacity and Family Planning

The analysis of statistical data on births and infant mortality has provided clear evidence of structures of social inequality. Differing processes of everyday life, such as those associated with rearing a

---

65. F.W.A. van Poppel's discussion of the case of the Netherlands is rich in

family and caring for and raising small children, are evidently shaped by a number of different factors which, though they can only be specified in detail in a small number of cases, can be said to create inequality. It is apparent that income — wealth in general, in fact — occupational status and thus, in Max Weber's words, the 'causal components of market situation', must be regarded as general indicators which can serve to identify a set of forces that cause the conditions and outcomes of everyday processes to vary among social groups. Although differing infant mortality rates and numbers of children per married couple show that these processes assume varying shapes and forms, there is no conclusive evidence to suggest that they are exclusively, or even unambiguously, determined by factors such as income, wealth, occupational status or associated levels of qualification (omitted from my own statistics). Under certain circumstances, other factors can come into play which are equally influential — or at least have a modifying effect — such as attitudes and patterns of behaviour related to sexuality, familial reproduction, infants' diets, the care of sick infants, the type of housing and living arrangements, the way the household's disposable income is spent, and the use of infrastructural services provided by the state or by charitable bodies. All of these are central elements of life style. The result, then, is an overlap between the effects of market capacity and traditional class attitudes on the one hand, and life styles, on the other, which, for analytical purposes, are regarded as pertaining to the level of social stratification.

I believe I have provided enough evidence to show that the process of social modernisation that accompanied industrialisation was reflected, from an early stage, in shifts in patterns of reproductive behaviour and in the conditions and consequences of producing and raising children. This long-term process, which accelerated in the lower classes after the First World War, led not only to rises in average living standards and to an overall increase in disposable life chances, which were expressed in the fall in the general infant mortality rate. More significantly, it also resulted, to varying degrees, in improvements in different spheres of society, and thus in different social groups. Although this process modified the traditional social order only in the upper and middle strata, it none the less created new forms in the distribution of actual life chances.

---

empirical data but lacks details of social differentiation: *Differential Fertility in the Netherlands: An Overview of Long-Term Trends with Special Reference to the Post-World War I Cohorts*, Working Paper no. 39, Netherlands Interuniversity Demographic Institute (Voorburg, 1983), pp. 21–9.

It is true that the relative positions of the middle and lower strata in the social hierarchy did not change significantly (they were certainly not reversed). However, while structures of relative distribution do appear to have remained constant, we should not forget the tangible changes which society was undergoing, and which were making themselves felt in the form of real opportunities and improved life chances.

For example, infant mortality rates, and the range of disposable life chances indicated by them, show that large sections of what are termed the middle classes managed to reach a privileged social position. Almost all the statistics I have included reflect the comparatively favourable chances their infants had of surviving. Middle-class parents practised forms of infant and child care that were, presumably, consistent with their interest in rational family planning, the success of which could be ensured by every child surviving. Similar attitudes began to be held not only by the elite group of graduate public officials and those in the liberal professions, but also by all sections of the 'new middle classes', albeit to varying degrees and at different stages. But in any case, these groups were all ahead of the mass of society in this respect.

A further undoubtedly important factor was that, during the course of the Wilhelmine Empire, interest groups and sections of the power elite pursued policies that were virtually designed to privilege the status groups of the 'new middle class'. Efforts to reform Prussian education during the 1880s and 1890s were particularly important in this respect.[66] They were sparked off by the notion of a 'qualification crisis', and led to a situation in which the educated middle classes established a privileged position within the education system. One should also note the campaign for the Insurance Laws on Salaried Employees (*Angestellten-Versicherungsgesetz*) during the early twentieth century, which had the effect of privileging white-collar workers, and thus of segregating them

---

66. See H.-G. Herrlitz and H. Titze, 'Überfüllung als bildungspolitische Strategie: Zur administrativen Steuerung der Lehrerarbeitslosigkeit in Preussen 1870–1914', *Die Deutsche Schule*, 68 (1976), pp. 348–70; D.K. Müller, 'Qualifikationskrise und Schulreform' in U. Herrmann (ed.), *Historische Pädagogik* (*Zeitschrift für Pädagogik*, supplement 14), (Weinheim und Basel, 1977), pp. 13–35; S.F. Müller, 'Mittelständische Schulpolitik, Die Rezeption des Überfüllungsproblems im gewerblichen und Bildungsbürgertum am Ende des 19. Jahrhunderts', *Historische Pädagogik*, pp. 79–97; H. Titze, 'Überfüllungskrisen in akademischen Karrieren: eine Zyklustheorie', *Zeitschrift für Pädagogik*, 27(2) (1981), pp. 187–224; idem, 'Enrolment Expansion and Academic Overcrowding in Germany' in K.H. Jarausch (ed.), *The Transformation of Higher Learning 1860–1930. Expansion, Diversification, Social Opening and Professionalization in England, Germany, Russia and the United States* (Stuttgart, 1983), pp. 57–88.

from the working class.[67] There were also at that time attempts to provide a form of privileged hospital care for middle-class patients.[68] All such measures aimed to improve middle-class access to the new kinds of institution that were enhancing or redistributing life chances in modern terms — higher education, improved health care and prevention of illness, social security against accidents, sickness or old age, and so on — in such a way that the opportunities the majority of the working classes had of benefiting from them were curtailed. This policy, by which certain privileges were established and others directly or indirectly excluded, was, however, ambivalent. On the one hand, it tended to undermine existing structures of inequality (that is, in the long term it improved the market capacity of the propertyless middle classes in relation to the propertied middle classes and above all to the aristocracy). On the other hand, in the political context of the latter years of the Empire it hindered the emancipation of the working-class population. None the less, it did have the effect of steering social modernisation in the direction of the welfarist infrastructure encountered in late capitalism. From this perspective, it can be concluded that by pursuing policies designed to grant them privilege or tending to exclude other social strata, the middle classes sought to consolidate the way in which components of the market capacity of certain social groups were being revalued in the wake of continuous industrialisation. Following Max Weber, we can say that phases of

67. See, for example, J. Kocka, 'Vorindustrielle Faktoren in der deutschen Industrialisierung. Industriebürokratie und "neuer Mittelstand" ' in M. Stürmer (ed.), *Das kaiserliche Deutschland* (Düsseldorf, 1970), pp. 275–8; idem, *Angestellte zwischen Faschismus und Demokratie. Zur politischen Sozialgeschichte der Angestellten: USA 1890–1940 im internationalen Vergleich*, vol. 25 of *Kritische Studien zur Geschichtswissenschaft* (Göttingen, 1977), pp. 48–52; U. Kadritzke, *Angestellte — Die geduldigen Arbeiter. Zur Soziologie und sozialen Bewegung der Angestellten* (Frankfurt an Main und Cologne, 1975), pp. 204–32, esp. 222–3. For a critique of the tendency Kocka has of regarding putative traditional orientations among the 'new middle class', particularly white-collar workers, as the source of strategies designed to bring privilege, and for a new approach to analysing the reproductive behaviour of white-collar workers, see R. Spree, 'Angestellte als Modernisierungsagenten: Indikatoren und Thesen zum reproduktiven Verhalten von Angestellten im späten 19. und frühen 20. Jahrhundert' in J. Kocka (ed.), *Angestellte Mittelschichten im 19. und 20. Jahrhundert im europäischen Vergleich*, special issue no. 7 of *Geschichte und Gesellschaft*, (Göttingen 1981), pp. 279–308.
68. A relevant example is given by the efforts of the middle classes from the beginning of the twentieth century onwards to establish special care facilities in general hospitals. They attempted to gain privileged treatment by demanding higher-quality care in separate hospital rooms with fewer patients, and at prices below the actual cost of the care. This was tantamount to asking for the middle classes to be subsidised and given preferential treatment at the expense of other patients who were dependent upon poor relief schemes and sickness insurance: see M. Stürzbecher, 'Aus der Diskussion über das "Klassenlose Krankenhaus" in Alt-Berlin', *Berliner Ärzteblatt*, 85 (10) (1972), pp. 509–21. For a contemporary view see *Das deutsche Reich in gesundheitlicher und demographisher Beziehung*.

accelerated technological and economic structural change initiate processes of class formation and, inevitably, revaluation of market capacities, while undermining traditional status positions.[69] From this perspective, it might be possible to conclude that in the last decade before the First World War, the middle classes found that during the previous decades of vigorous economic modernisation central components of their market capacity (i.e. qualifications in the broadest sense) had been enhanced. Partially supported by the power elites, the aim of the middle classes was to convert this situation into one enabling them, as status groups, to occupying positions fixed in the social structure. In particular, this meant that the mass of the working class, which itself was beginning to proceed along similar lines, had to be subjugated within the social hierarchy, especially with regard to education and the health system.

Of course these conclusions are speculative in character and rather overstretch the documentary evidence available. Even if we argue on a less theoretical level, it remains true that infrastructural developments (for instance, urban sanitation, improvements in hospitals and the education system) should not be regarded simply as vehicles for providing more equal opportunities among the major social classes and strata. We should bear in mind, for example, that in some cases access to educational institutions was restricted, which only emphasised the existing disparities in wealth and income. Moreover, it should not be forgotten that not every group was aware of (possibly fatal) dangers to health, nor of how to avoid them, nor of how to improve their situation by taking advantage of infrastructural facilities. It is likely that, compared with the working classes for instance, the 'new middle class' had acquired to a much greater degree the kind of experience and knowledge which is needed when dealing with public institutions. The equalisation of all classes by, as it were, 'blind fate' — in the form of disease and death among infants, infections in adulthood, large numbers of unwanted children, and so on — was reversed, especially in the middle classes. Although the infrastructure was supposed to be open to all social groups, I subscribe to the view that initially it was primarily the 'new middle class' which was able to benefit most from such services and make access to them more

---

69. See M. Weber, *Wirtschaft und Gesellschaft. Grundriß der verstehenden Soziologie*, 5th revised edn (Tübingen, 1972), pp. 538–9. F. Ringer develops further the Weberian idea of the connection between economic and social structure in the concrete historical context in *Education and Society in Modern Europe* (Bloomington, IN and London, 1979), pp. 12–22.

difficult for others, if not by establishing formal regulations then at least by engaging in some form of propaganda.

The unequal distribution of life chances which was in evidence among the working class can be attributed to three main factors: the growing disparity between urban and rural living standards and working conditions; the growth in the numbers of people with professional qualifications; and the widespread assimilation of the forms of action and social behaviour typical of a modern urban industrial society (reflected *inter alia* in party or trade union membership). These factors were important components in the process by which everyday life became rationalised. In general, infant mortality rates and the average numbers of children were lower among blue-collar workers in the secondary sector than among those in the primary. A comparison of the secondary and tertiary sectors also shows that the corresponding figures in the latter were lower, though in this case they were less marked. Such disparities can be seen even more clearly if they are measured with respect to differing levels of qualification (in the present study this could only be deduced indirectly from membership of a particular trade or profession). The three factors we have mentioned converged to a certain degree, inasmuch as a higher level of professional training was often related to greater political involvement, and both of these depended on the greatest possible degree of integration into the urban industrial environment. As a result, changes occurred at differing speeds and to varying degrees in the different sections of the working class, with all these strata lagging behind the 'new middle class'.

Part of the reason why such changes occurred at varying times is connected with the particular conditions of work and everyday life in different classes of dependent wage earners. In the sphere of production (i.e. in the area which was central to social strategy), considerable obstacles stood in the way of workers who consciously attempted to structure their own social environment — this was particularly the case before 1914 when trade unions were not permitted to form a legal part of Germany's political and economic landscape. At the same time, however, sections of the working class, in the first instance the skilled (organised) workers, were creating greater scope for action within the sphere of reproduction. This found particular expression in the transition to family planning and birth control. The modernisation and industrialisation of German society was being shaped by a general process of rationalisation which, we may suppose, was no longer being accepted passively as an inevitable outcome of the conditions of production (in the form of intensified pressure to work and perform). Around the turn of the century, individuals were beginning actively to incorporate the process into the way they structured their lives. As an element shaping individual life styles, the rationalisation of everyday life, particularly of patterns of human reproduction, acted as an important mechanism which provided a reduction of social constraint (caused by cramped resources) and opened up new opportunities, as can be seen in the fall in the infant mortality rate.

As time passed, the figures for our two key indicators (infant mortality and the number of children per married couple) in the 'new middle class' and in sections of the working class gradually began to converge. At least the general trends suggest that this was the case. Nevertheless, the function of the rationalisation of reproductive behaviour which this implies was different in each social group because of the varying strains imposed by different working environments and the average disposable economic resources (i.e. as a result of different market capacities). Put simply and rather stereotypically, among the 'new middle class', rational behaviour meant that the educated strata were able to meet the norms of consumption commensurate with their status group, and the strata of non-graduate public officials and white-collar workers were able to achieve the upward social mobility they desired (through investing in the education of their children and/or by accumulating status symbols). In equally crude terms, it might be said that for the working class, the rationalisation of life functioned initially as a way of ensuring minimal benefits from material social progress and the basic physical survival of the members of the family. Thus the notion that the 'new middle class' were the harbingers of the introduction of birth control (a thesis proposed by Adelheid von Nell)[70] is true only in a chronological sense. Even then, this idea still presents some problems because it assumes that the size of the average middle-class family was the norm. However, from the point of view of social history, the decisive factor is not whether family sizes became more uniform, but the *extent* to which they had changed within each social group when compared with the situation at the beginning of the period under discussion. In this respect, the changes among farmers were particularly radical. The same was true of the working class, though there was a delay of one or two generations when compared with the 'new middle classes'. It is probable that the shifts in attitudes that this entailed were mediated extremely indirectly by changes in the social structure, without

70. See von Nell, 'Die Entwicklung', pp. 15–16, 119ff.

certain middle-class groups functioning as a kind of model or norm.

Finally, it should be noted that in my view the greater importance of rationality in people's lives, and to this extent of family planning and birth control (and by rationality I mean a growing awareness of the ability to mould one's own fate and break with traditional, fatalistic and above all religious and mystical notions of normal behaviour) by no means necessarily implies that the number of children born to a married couple was to be reduced at any price and in every social situation. This particular interpretation of modernity is, rather, consistent with an observation that was made with regard to the families of white-collar workers shortly before the First World War and which has been confirmed on repeated occasions ever since: families in the low-income bracket deliberately introduced birth control to reduce the number of births, while as income levels increased there was a proportional increase in the number of births and thus in family size.[71]

---

71. See A Günther,'Die deutschen Techniker', *Soziale Praxis und Archiv für Volkswohlfahrt*, 21 (20/21), (1911–12), pp. 674–5; idem, *Lebenshaltung des Mittelstandes. Statistische und theoretische Untersuchungen zur Konsumtionslehre*, vol. 146/2 of Schriften des Vereins für Socialpolitik (Munich and Leipzig, 1920), p. 21. For a more differentiated approach which attempts to interpret differences in patterns of consumption as indicators of diverse mentalities and life styles, see S. Coyner, 'Class Consciousness and Consumption: The New Middle Class during the Weimar Republic', *Journal of Social History*, 10 (3) (1977); idem, 'Class Patterns of Family Income and Expenditure during the Weimar Republic: German White-Collar Employees as Harbingers of Modern Society', (Unpublished PhD thesis, Rutgers University, New Brunswick, NJ, 1975) pp. 107, 393; Spree, 'Angestellte als Modernisierungsagenten'.

Part II
Determinants of the Decline in Mortality

In the first part of this book, I set out to describe the changes that took place in health and mortality in the German population between 1871 and 1914, concentrating initially on a set of systematically interdependent indicators that I applied to that total population. Even in the early stages of the analysis, considerable emphasis was placed on the important variations with respect to sex, age, size of population, region, disease or cause of death, which differentiated the overall trends. Limiting the analysis to infant and child mortality, the socio-structural implications of all these deviations were then considered in more detail, and a number of intervening variables were discussed. I repeatedly referred to the wider social environment in which the processes of social differentiation caused by changing patterns in sickness and health actually occurred. The differences between the levels of health and mortality in the various social groups may be interpreted, to a certain extent, as the result of an unequal distribution of marketable resources (market capacity). However, as the health sector and the health-related social infrastructure proceeded to expand, a situation arose in which market-bound life chances could be redistributed. Indeed, this almost certainly took place during the period under discussion. In the preceding section I began to discuss the fact that the ability to make the best possible use of these social and medical services and infrastructural facilities is closely tied to certain preconditions which are divided unequally in society. The extent to which these facilities are used is not influenced simply by information — awareness or knowledge — nor even by the actual availability of such services. It is also affected by traditional patterns of social behaviour and attitudes peculiar to a social group. In order to be able to compare and contrast in some meaningful way the importance of market forces, on the one hand, and social attitudes, on the other, for the development of health and mortality, we shall have to assess in more detail the changes in the social environment which formed the framework for developments in the 'people's health'.

The underlying trend that is visible in the changes that affected health and mortality between 1870 and 1914 was an improvement in average life expectancy (or, alternatively, a fall in the mortality rates) in all age groups, and with regard to virtually all of the major fatal diseases. Nothing seems more obvious, or corresponds more to the opinion that doctors and lay people alike have been expressing for 70–80 years, than to conclude that these developments can be attributed to the quantitative expansion of and qualitative improvements in the health sector.[1] Even the tendency mentioned above for the health of a working man or woman — especially one from the urban working classes — to deteriorate later on in his or her working life, does not cast doubt on the correctness of such a conclusion. In view of the greater stresses and strains that had been a feature of the various trades and industries since the beginning of the industrialisation process and the acute housing shortage, which actually worsened during this period — especially in the towns and cities — it would be reasonable to maintain that if the health sector had not been dramatically expanded, the state of the 'people's health' would in fact have become even worse than the indicators suggest. Strictly speaking, then, the questions that this prompts call for a systematic causal analysis. However, I am not in a position to do exactly that because of the inadequacy of my own knowledge and lack of time and energy — not to mention the complex nature of the subject-matter, which is only one part of the process of profound social changes that had been taking place since the beginnings of industrialisation. Instead I shall follow McKeown's examples and concentrate on no more than a few aspects of this process (development of the health sector and health-related infrastructure and changes in real income levels and dietary patterns). Contemporary observers, and the most eminent specialists since then, have acknowledged that these factors deeply affect the nature of changes in mortality rates and standards of health. It is never the notion that such influences exist, but their relative strengths that are disputed.

1. For a contemporary view, see, for example, Kirchner, 'Die Seuchenbekämpfung unter Berücksichtigung der einschlägigen deutschen und preußischen Gesetzgebung', and Aschenborn, 'Ärzte', both in O. Rapmund (ed.), *Das Preußische Medizinal- und Gesundheitswesen in den Jahren 1883–1908. Festschrift zur Feier des 25 jährigen Bestehens des Preußischen Medizinalbeamten-Vereins* (Berlin, 1908), pp. 196–7, 352–3; O.v. Bollinger, *Wandlungen der Medizin und des Ärztestandes in den letzten 50 Jahren* (Munich, 1909), pp. 40–1. Vor dem Esche, for example, is somewhat more cautious, but basically convinced that the expansion of doctors' services was of 'causal significance' for the fall in mortality and in the incidence of infectious diseases: 'Die Verbreitung der Ärzte im Deutschen Reich bzw. in der Bundesrepublik von 1876–1950, *Archiv für Hygiene, 138* (1954), p. 374. In the literature of medical history and of demography, it is a matter of controversy whether the expansion of health care in the late nineteenth and early twentieth centuries in the states of Central and Western Europe did in fact manage to have any significant impact on life chances related to health and a higher life expectancy. See the literature cited on p. 8, n. 2.

One example of the problems this can cause is raised by Preston in his comprehensive study of the long-term changes in mortality that have taken place in 165 population groups from 43 nations over the last 100 years.[2] Preston is critical of McKeown's hypotheses, which claim that neither medical science, the therapeutic skill of doctors, nor the institutions of the health sector in the narrower sense had much influence on the fall in the mortality rates in England and Wales during the nineteenth century. Preston is convinced that this fall was brought about by a whole range of different factors: developments and improvements in antiseptic techniques; measures taken to isolate illnesses by putting victims in quarantine; the monitoring and purification of food and water; improvements in sanitation, personal hygiene and, in particular, child nutrition; and, finally, the development of specifically therapeutic medical remedies. Every one of these factors — and in Preston's view this is a decisive point — was a direct consequence of the developments and successes in the field of bacteriology and thus of the progress made in medical science.[3] Preston therefore does not merely simply list a number of factors and examine their historical significance, as McKeown does. His arguments are more sharply focused than McKeown's for the simple reason that he traces these factors back to a single common cause: advances in bacteriology.

In the following chapters I shall discuss, from a specifically German perspective, a number of these factors that, according to Preston and others, had a bearing on the fall in the mortality rates. Unfortunately, there is very little relevant literature on the subject to fall back on here. For although the amount of literature which contained a whole range of opinions on this subject grew at a steady rate after the turn of the century, there is a shortage of reliable empirical evidence. Perhaps the most serious failing is the lack of a well-argued comparison of all the various relevant factors.[4] Exceptions to this are the studies by Lee and Dickler.[5] However, the

---

2. See Preston, *Mortality Patterns*, pp. 3–4.
3. Idem, pp. 42ff and 81–2.
4. See, for example, Grotjahn, *Soziale Pathologie*, pp. 44ff, 50ff, 449–50; Prinzing, *Handbuch*, 2nd edn, p. 474, 482ff, 513ff; idem, 'Die Gesundheitsstatistik', pp. 40ff; H. Kaupen-Haas, 'Gesundheitsverhalten und Krankheitsverhalten aus historischer Sicht. Zwei Strategien zur Gesundheitssicherung' in *Jahrbuch für kritische Medizin*, vol. 1 (Berlin, 1976), pp. 86–100.
5. Lee, 'Germany', pp. 149–58; idem, 'The Mechanism of Mortality Change in Germany, 1750–1850', *Medizinhistorisches Journal*, 15(3) (1980), pp. 244–68; R. A. Dickler, 'Labor Market Pressure Aspects of Agricultural Growth in the Eastern Region of Prussia, 1840–1914: A Case Study of Economic-Demographic Interrelations during the Demographic Transition' (unpubl. diss., University of Pennsylvania, 1975), pp. 152–217. See also Abholz, 'Welche Bedeutung hat die Medizin'. For an original approach, see F.B. Smith, *The People's Health 1830–1910* (London,

former restricts himself to a general outline, and the latter concentrates on the Eastern provinces of Prussia, arriving at conclusions concerning the possible effects both of the expansion of the health sector and — to an even greater extent — the expansion of the infrastructure that are not always convincing. My own analysis proceeds from Lee's conclusion that debate about reasons for the decline in the mortality rates in Germany remains far from closed because the data available do not provide enough conclusive evidence to vindicate any of the better-known hypotheses.[6] However, if this whole question could be placed in a more systematic context, and additional empirical evidence examined, then it seems to me that it might be possible to compare the plausibility of these different hypotheses. Such an approach would enable us to weigh up the various factors in this controversy more clearly. Of course, this particular accent to my investigation is not intended to replace a more strictly logical causal analysis but will, I hope, render it easier to explain the problems we have touched on here.

The question of whether the changes in the level of public health referred to above were influenced in any significant way by the expansion of the health sector will be to the fore in the following analysis. In this context, I shall also discuss any additional or alternative influences, and I shall devote more attention than is usual in such studies to the phenomena of regional and social inequality. This will make it possible to shed light on aspects of the redistribution of life chances that resulted from the expansion of the infrastructure. Moreover, I shall occasionally assess the relative stability of, and the changes in, structures of social inequality, so as to be able to judge the impact of each of the factors determining the average level of public health.

1979), while a review of the literature is given by A. Labisch, 'Sozialgeschichte der Medizin. Methodologische Überlegungen und Forschungsbericht', *Archiv für Sozialgeschichte,* 20 (1980), pp. 431–69. In addition, F. Rothenbacher compiles relevant statistical data in 'Die Entwicklung der Gesundheitsverhältnisse in Deutschland seit der Industrialisierung' in E. Wiegand and W. Zapf (eds), *Wandel der Lebensbedingungen in Deutschland. Wohlfahrtsentwicklung seit der Industrialisierung* (Frankfurt am Main and New York, 1982), pp. 335–94.

6. See Lee, 'Germany', p. 158.

3
The Expansion of the Health Sector

At this point I should attempt to define more precisely what I actually mean by the already frequently used term 'health sector'. In the following sections, health sector will be used to refer to the sum total of people, institutions and material resources that are specifically designated to preserve, protect or restore the health of the individual and minimise the effects of sickness or other kinds of affliction.[7] The services and social developments that affect the human environment, rather than the individual directly, by means of changes in the material and institutional environment, are regarded as separate from the health sector and are referred to as the 'health-related infrastructure'. At the same time it will be assumed that the effectiveness of the services provided by the health authorities generally presupposes a minimum level of co-operation and initiative on the part of the individual.

This definition of both the producer and consumer aspects of the health sector may appear to be a little over-restrictive for the purposes of an historical investigation such as this, but it does make it possible to structure more clearly the complex web of relationships within which changes in the patterns of sickness and health took place. I shall therefore abide by this distinction between a specifically functional health sector, on the one hand, and a multi-functional, yet health-related infrastructure, on the other. The criterion used to distinguish between them concerns, therefore, not just the function they are designed to fulfil, but also, above all, the differences in the way that access to them is regulated: for whilst the use of health-sector facilities is generally regulated on an individual basis, and generally depends on some form of direct payment by the individual concerned, the services provided by the health-related infrastructure benefit large groups of people in a number of sometimes extremely diverse ways and are 'paid for' on a more collective basis by means of public taxation.

---

7. See Kohn and White, *Health Care*, p. 3.

3.1 Evidence of Quantitative Changes

The following sections will be concerned with indicators that refer to two areas: the quantitative aspect of the facilities provided by the health sector, and their qualitative aspect. Each of these two aspects will be described from a number of different perspectives, including, on occasion, the perspectives of regional or social inequality. However, I shall begin by presenting statistical evidence that there was an expansion of the services available. A frequently cited indicator in this respect is the number of doctors. If this term is meant to refer to a professional group with clearly demarcated function — in other words to those people who are regularly asked for help in cases of sickness or imminent death, or who give advice on ways of staying healthy and avoiding sickness — then it is even more difficult to establish the boundaries of this group for the period under analysis than would be the case even today. A closer examination of the group that fulfils these functions will reveal that, even in our own highly industrialised and enlightened society, it is not at all identical with the actual number of qualified and registered doctors. It is in fact much greater. For quite apart from *bona fide* medical doctors, Western society today is also able to accommodate state-certified non-medical practitioners and qualified or unqualified psychotherapists, not to mention the large numbers of other individuals who, either professionally or on a part-time basis, provide advice or health care for the sick. Within the context of the period under discussion, one particularly important development was the promulgation of the Trade Acts (*Gewerbeordnungen*) in 1869 and 1871, which went so far as to classify medicine as a free trade and thus immediately created a two-tier system of health-care. On the one hand, there was the body of university-trained doctors specialising in various fields who were constantly pressing for greater standardisation, especially in state-approved education and training, and in various forms of examinations. On the other, whole areas of advice and health care were left to groups of people whose training and practical experience as consultants and healers had not been subject to any form of specific official control. The members of this second group were constantly being dismissed as 'charlatans', 'quacks' and so on by doctors and their professional association.[8]

8. See C. Huerkamp, 'Ärzte und Professionalisierung in Deutschland. Überlegungen zum Wandel des Arztberufs im 19. Jahrhundert', *Geschichte und Gesellschaft*, 6(3) (1980), pp. 349–82; also Gottstein, *Das Heilwesen der Gegenwart* (Berlin, 1924), pp. 311ff, who, in fact, takes a fairly moderate line on lay medicine;

Determinants of the Decline in Mortality

None the less, in the light of more recent experience with the failings of scientific professional medicine, on the one hand, and, on the other, with the advantages that can be gained from various forms of lay or alternative medicine (such as naturopathy, psychosomatic medicine and depth psychology, etc.) that have arisen out of a wide range of bodies of knowledge and traditions, it would be erroneous simply to assume that the doctors were the only ones who contributed to the improvements in the 'people's health' during the Wilhelmine Empire. It should not be forgotten that, in many rural areas in particular, there was an old tradition of relying in the first instance on time-honoured 'household remedies' if someone became ill and then of seeking the advice of a whole series of 'healers' from the surrounding area (such as 'wise old women', shepherds, faith-healers, 'sorcerers' and barber-surgeons, etc.). Only then, perhaps, would people approach the priest or, possibly, the village schoolteacher.[9] It was only if all else failed that they would seek out a doctor, who usually lived some distance away in the next town (I shall return to this problem in Part III below).

If I none the less resort to doctors as the most important indicator of the number of people active in the health sector, this is because their numbers have been recorded more or less accurately, which — not surprisingly in view of the foregoing — is not true of the other types of healer. In 1876 there were 13,728 doctors in the German Empire. By 1900, the figure had risen to 27,374 and, by 1913, to 34,136. This suggests that the corresponding service available doubled between 1876 and 1900 and rose by a further 50 per cent between 1900 and 1913. The growth rate therefore accelerated rapidly towards the end of the nineteenth century and at the beginning of the twentieth. The improvement in the numbers of doctors per head of population was less impressive, however. This

---

and K.E. Rothschuh, *Naturheilbewegung, Reformbewegung, Alternativbewegung* (Stuttgart, 1983). For a recent and comprehensive account of the whole question of the professionalisation of medicine and of the development of the doctor–patient relationship, see C. Huerkamp, *Der Aufstieg der Ärzte im 19. Jahrhundert. Vom gelehrten Stand zum professionellen Experten. Das Beispiel Preussens* (Göttingen, 1985); E. Shorter, *Bedside Manners. The Troubled History of Doctors and Patients* (New York, 1985).

9. See Gottstein, *Das Heilwesen*, pp. 312–13; H. Pompey, 'Pastoralmedizin — der Beitrag der Seelsorge zur psycho-physischen Gesundheit' in Imhof, *Mensch und Gesundheit; Das Gesundheitswesen des Preußischen Staates im Jahre 1901*, p. 493; indicative of the 'modern' approach to the problem is R. Schenda, 'Das Verhalten der Patienten im Schnittpunkt professionalisierter und naiver Gesundheitsversorgung' in M Blohmke et al. (eds), *Handbuch der Sozialmedizin, vol. 3: Sozialmedizin in der Praxis* (Stuttgart, 1976), pp. 31–45. Here lay medicine and medical self-help are discussed using the value-laden term 'subcultural health attitudes to health'.

rose from 3.2 doctors to every 10,000 people in 1876 to 4.9 in 1900, but by 1913 had only reached 5.1. Thus, compared with the rate of population growth, the number of doctors grew much more slowly in the course of the last 20 years of the period under analysis — especially after 1900 (the background to these developments will also be discussed in greater detail in Chapter 10 below).[10]

In view of the fact that even as late as 1913 each doctor was responsible for an average of approximately 2000 people and an area of 15 square km, it is apparent that, despite the rapid growth in the number of doctors and the amount of treatment available, by 1914 the level of medical care had become no more than moderate. It is also worth noting that these averages obscure a broad range of regional variation. The trend was towards a greater concentration of doctors in the industrialised conurbations and towns than in the rural, agricultural areas, which lagged some way behind. After 1900 in particular, the range separating the regions with highest and lowest numbers of doctors per head of population widened considerably (see Table 18). A series of statistical tests, which I use to examine the relative percentages of doctors per head of population in each region, confirms this impression, but also suggests that a minor qualification is necessary. It seems to have been the case that the differences in the levels of medical care available in each region increased considerably in absolute terms, whereas their relative positions in this hierarchy remained unchanged right up to 1914. Although the rural, agricultural regions were disadvantaged in this way, new patterns of social inequality were not created: traditional ones were merely consolidated.[11] Moreover, the figures for the level of medical care are misleading because the doctors' role in

10. Taken from vor dem Esche, *Die Verbreitung der Ärzte*, pp. 374, 381; M.Stürzbecher, 'Die medizinische Versorgung und die Entstehung der Gesundheitsfürsorge zu Beginn des 20. Jahrhunderts in Deutschland' in G. Mann and R. Winau (eds), *Medizin, Naturwissenschaft, Technik und das Zweite Kaisserreich* (Göttingen, 1977), pp. 240–1, 251–7.

11. For example, between 1876 and 1909 in the Prussian provinces, the variation coefficient (which can be used to measure inequality) of the number of licensed doctors per 10,000 inhabitants did not vary significantly. There is evidence to suggest that even the introduction of statutory sickness insurance failed to bring about any meaningful change in existing structures: the correlation between the number of those covered by sickness insurance and doctors in each Prussian province was as high in 1887, i.e. at a time when the insurance legislation could hardly have had any impact, as it was in 1909 (in 1887, $r = 0.94$; in 1909, $r = 0.92$). While this might be indicative of a general trend, the units of analysis — Prussian provinces — are somewhat too large to allow reliable conclusions to be drawn about distribution. For similar conclusions see K. Borchardt, 'Regionale Wachstumsdifferenzierung in Deutschland im 19. Jahrhundert unter besonderer Berücksichtigung des West-Ost-Gefälles' in W. Abel et. al. (eds), *Wirtschaft, Geschichte und Wirtschaftsgeschichte. Festschrift zum 65. Geburtstag von Friedrich Lütge* (Stuttgart, 1966), pp. 336, 339.

giving practical advice on health and treating the sick varied considerably, depending on which region and social group was involved. The numbers of people who claimed to 'practise medicine professionally' but who were not licensed by the state ('quacks'), which local medical officers in Prussia had begun to record in 1902, are appropriate indicators of this. Since such 'quacks' were under no obligation to register with the authorities, the published figures of the number of people who came into this category must have been extremely approximate. And since, moreover, it may be assumed that there were considerable deficiencies in the information collected by the district medical officers (presumably, many of the acts of 'quackery' were conducted in secret by those involved), these figures should not be taken too seriously. None the less, it is quite clear that this particular group was indeed strongly represented in Prussia, its number growing from 5,148 in 1903 to 5,610 in 1913, despite persecution and a series of other measures taken by the medical profession to suppress them.[12] Compared with the numbers of fully qualified doctors available (18,219 in 1903 and 20,394 in 1913), the percentage of 'quacks' in Prussia remained at a virtually constant 28 per cent from 1903 to 1913 (see Table 19).

A look at the figures for each of the administrative districts will demonstrate their random quality. All the same, they still convey some idea of the actual importance of alternative forms of medicine for health care. Greater Berlin alone counted over 1000 trading 'quacks' in both 1903 and 1913 (though this amounted to no more than a third of the number of doctors). In the district of Frankfurt an der Oder, 302 'quacks' were recorded in 1903, which was around 75 per cent of the number of doctors in this area — a proportion that corresponded to that in the administrative district of Köslin, where there were 117 known 'quacks' in 1903. Although these figures varied considerably in individual cases, there is a clear trend which suggests that 'quacks' were much more important in the Eastern, rural provinces of Prussia than in the West. In the administrative district of Arnsberg, for example, there were no

12. Gottstein suspects that there was a large rise in the number of lay healers, particularly during the last two decades of the nineteenth century, and that this was greatly underestimated in all the official statistics. See Gottstein, *Das Heilwesen*, pp. 312–13. Figures are taken from: *Das Gesundheitswesen des Preußischen Staates im Jahre 1903* (Berlin, 1905), pp. 437ff; *Das Gesundheitswesen des Preußischen Staates im Jahre 1913*, pp. 467–8. For more detail see R. Spree, 'Kurpfuscherei-Bekämpfung und ihre sozialen Funktionen während des 19. und zu Beginn des 20. Jahrhunderts'in A. Labisch and R. Spree (eds), *Medizin und sozialez Wandel* (Bonn, 1988). A more thorough account which deals only with England is J. Woodward and D. Richards (eds), *Health Care and Popular Medicine in Nineteenth-Century England: Essays in the History of Medicine* (London, 1977).

more than 36 known 'quacks' in 1903, which was around 4 per cent of the total number of doctors. Because these figures are of necessity so imprecise, they do not go very far towards confirming our perception of the levels of medical care provided in the different regions and social groups during the period under discussion. However, while they do indicate that the growth in the numbers of doctors reflects the trend towards a growing professionalisation of the health sector, they do not seem to be suitable for assessing the exact nature of the changes in the intensity of medical care available to large sections of the population. For whilst the number of 'quacks' known to district medical officers seems to suggest that there were two to three doctors for every lay practitioner, the actual relationship was probably the reverse, especially in rural communities.

A second quantitative aspect of the available medical facilities that was probably even more important, at least in the long term, was the expansion of the hospital service between 1871 and 1914. Here, too, problems arise in distinguishing between public, private and university hospitals, on the one hand, and the large general hospitals and the more specialised clinics for psychiatric disorders, eye clinics and maternity hospitals, on the other. For various practical reasons, we shall concentrate our attention on the general hospitals, and take the number of beds as an indication of the service provided. These were first reliably recorded for the whole of the German Empire in 1877, when there were 72,219 beds, a figure which had risen to 226,831 by 1911.[13] Thus, during this period, the number of beds available in general hospitals had increased by almost 300 per cent. It should also be noted that between 1900 and 1911 almost the same number of new beds, approximately 100,000, were made available as for the period from 1877 to 1900. Thus, although the number of doctors increased moderately during the first decade of this century, the number of hospital beds rose dramatically. The number of beds per head of population also improved, from 16.5 per 10,000 people in 1877 to 41.5 in 1911. Adding all the different types of hospital together, the relative

13. From vor dem Esche, 'Die Versorgung der Bevölkerung mit Krankenhäusern', pp. 387–8; Stürzbecher, 'Die medizinische Versorgung', pp. 249, 258. D. Jetter proceeds further in *Grundzüge der Krankenhausgeschichte (1800–1900)* (Darmstadt, 1977); A. Labisch, 'Das Krankenhaus in der Gesundheitspolitik der deutschen Sozialdemokratie vor dem Ersten Weltkrieg', *Medizinsoziologisches Jahrbuch*, 1 (1981), pp. 126–51; idem, 'Ärzte und Arbeiterbewegung', *Medizinsoziologische Mitteilungen*, 3(4) (1977), pp. 6–19. For a bibliography of works on the history of hospitals in Germany, among which there are very few socio-historical accounts, see *Historia Hospitalium. Zeitschrift der Deutschen Gesellschaft für Krankenhausgeschichte*, 13 (1979–1980), pp. 230–7.

number of beds available rose from 24.5 per 10,000 people in 1877 to 69.0 in 1913.

The introduction of statutory sickness insurance in 1883 may be regarded as an additional quantitative aspect of the medical facilities available. Quite apart from the effect this presumably had on working-class patterns of behaviour (see Part III below), this compulsory insurance must also be credited, above all, with stimulating the rise in the number of doctors and hospital beds.[14] The usual yardstick for the range of facilities covered by statutory sickness insurance is generally considered to be the number of members of the insurance schemes. This rose from 4.294 million in 1885 to 13.566 million in 1913. In 1885, 9.2 per cent of the total population of the German Empire were covered by statutory sickness insurance; by 1913 the figure had increased to just over 20 per cent (Table 20). Of course, these national averages obscure the considerable amount of regional and social variation in the membership of sickness insurance funds, as Table 20 indicates: in the heavily industrialised areas and large towns the percentage of people insured was far higher than the national average, while in rural areas it tended to be some way below it. A significant failing in the statistics is that there is no indication of the extent to which insurance funds were prepared to provide for the families of members as well as the members themselves. Any attempt to determine the numbers of people involved relies essentially on guesswork, or on specific surveys conducted by individual cities or insurance funds. Thus, in 1900 approximately 32,000 out of Augsburg population of 85,000 were legally insured (i.e. 37.4 per cent). Despite the fact that only a few of the insurance companies also covered other family members, this figure rises to 61 per cent if all others covered by the statutory funds are included.[15] In the course of an inquiry on sickness

---

14. On the establishment and development of sickness insurance, and for statistical data, see G.A. Ritter, *Social Welfare in Germany and Britain* (Leamington Spa, 1985); P.A. Köhler and H.F. Zacher (eds), *Beiträge zur Geschichte und aktueller Situation der Sozialversicherung* (Berlin, 1983); J. Alber, *Vom Armenhaus zum Wohlfahrtsstaat. Analysen zur Entwicklung der Sozialversicherung in Westeuropa* (Frankfurt am Main and New York, 1982); W.J. Mommsen and W. Mock (eds), *The Origins of the Welfare State in Britain and Germany* (London, 1982); P.A. Köhler and H.F. Zacher, *Ein Jahrhundert Sozialversicherung in der Bundesrepublik Deutschland, Frankreich, Großbritannien, Österreich, und der Schweiz* (Berlin, 1981); F. Tennstedt, *Sozialgeschichte der Sozialpolitik in Deutschland. Vom 18. Jahrhundert bis zum Ersten Weltkrieg* (Göttingen, 1981); idem, 'Sozialgeschichte der Sozialversicherung' in Blohmke et al., *Handbuch der Sozialmedizin*, pp. 385–492; H.-G. Reuter, 'Verteilungs- und Umverteilungseffekte der Sozialversicherungsgesetzgebung im Kaiserreich' in Blaich, *Staatliche Umverteilungspolitik*, pp. 107–63.
15. *Der ärztliche Stand und die deutsche Arbeiterversicherung. Aus Anlaß der bevorstehenden Abänderung des Krankenversicherungsgesetzes zusammengestellt vom ärztlichen Lokalverein Augsburg* (Augsburg, 1901), pp. 361–3.

insurance in 1896, doctors' representative councils in the province of Silesia managed to determine the extent of family sickness insurance. Their results indicated that in that province, 25 per cent of the insurance funds which insured 40 per cent of all insurance fund members, also provided free medical treatment for family dependants. In this respect, the administrative district of Oppeln was far more advanced, however: the dependants of 72.2 per cent of all those insured received free medical treatment. Assuming the average member had two or three others in the family, the total number of people in the area covered by statutory insurance grows from 639,629 (members only) to 1,286,346 (members plus insured dependants). Similarly, the corresponding increase in the percentage of the Silesian population that was insured rose from 14.7 per cent to 29.5 per cent, and in the administrative district of Oppeln from 14.3 per cent to as much as 40 per cent.[16] A more accurate study of the percentage of the population that was insured in each city throughout Germany would undoubtedly produce figures that in some cases would be even higher. However, the disparities were too great to make it worthwhile calculating an average figure. On balance, then, all that can be assumed is that, in some regions at least, the number of people provided with medical care was considerably higher than the 20 per cent that is suggested by the overall level of sickness insurance in the Reich.

3.2 Changes in the Quality of Care

Having discussed the quantitative improvements in the services provided by the health sector it is now time to examine the qualitative changes. The problem here, however, seems to be choosing a suitable set of indicators. The ideal type of indicator would enable us to assess the performance and output of the health

16. 'Ergebnisse der Enquête, nach denen die Prozentsätze ausgerechnet wurden', *Ärztliches Vereinsblatt für Deutschland* (hereafter *ÄVB*), 411 (1899), pp. 469–76; a summary is given in *Statistik des Deutschen Reichs*, new series, vol. 140: *Die Krankenversicherung im Jahre 1900* (Berlin, 1903), pp. 23–4. A similar investigation into the Administrative District of Cologne in 1904 concluded that the dependents of about one quarter of members of sickness insurance funds were also eligible for free medical treatment. Tennstedt, 'Sozialgeschichte der Sozialversicherung', p. 388, estimates that in 1913, counting individuals and the members of their families also covered, 50 per cent of the entire population of the Reich had sickness insurance. For a detailed account see C. Huerkamp and R. Spree, 'Arbeitsmarktstrategien der deutschen Ärzteschaft im späten 19. und frühen 20. Jahrhundert. Zur Entwicklung des Marktes für professionelle ärztliche Dienstleistungen in T. Pierenkemper and R.H. Tilly (eds), *Historische Arbeitsmarktforschung* (Göttingen, 1982), pp. 77–120, esp. pp. 93–103.

sector with a great degree of precision. In fact, efforts are being made in all branches of social science to produce such social indicators, but it is in the area of health that there has been least success. This is particularly true if these indicators are supposed to be obtained mainly from official statistics, since the latter almost exclusively record input (especially in the form of income or expenditure), rather than output. There are undoubtedly problems associated with the indicators selected here, but they are still felt to be useful within the contemporary debate. One of these is the average number of days spent by each patient in hospital per year. In 1877 the average for general hospitals came to 33.3 days. It then stagnated at a level of around 30 days until 1901, only to fall once again, this time to 28 days, shortly before the First World War.[17] Thus, in the course of the period under investigation, the average length of in-patient treatment in general hospitals fell by five days or around 16 per cent. One possible interpretation is that this fall reflects an improvement in the quality of in-patient care, inasmuch as illnesses were cured more quickly. However, in isolation, this single indicator — which, in addition, is all too easy to manipulate — is simply not sufficient to enable us to make a reliable judgement. The same applies to the second indicator of quality, the proportion of time that each bed was being used per year. In 1877, for example, the beds were only occupied for 51 per cent of the time in general hospitals, but by 1901 this figure had already risen to 60 per cent and 65 per cent by 1911. This indicates that the total number of days in which hospital treatment was administered had increased at a faster rate than the number of beds, with the result that the utilisation rate of hospital beds increased by about 18 per cent between 1877 and 1901, and an additional 9 per cent between 1901 and 1911. Most importantly, however, this indicator is rather a measure of efficiency, which underlines the fact that during the Wilhelmine Empire a surplus was created in the hospital service which increased in the 1890s and took a long time to reduce. It is however, only an indirect indicator of an improvement in hospital care since it can be maintained that as more people began to hear of the successes of treatment, there was such a growth in public demand that the number of 'surplus' beds was reduced.

One further indication of quality that is commonly used in modern health statistics is the number of medical personnel per hospital bed, a factor that is supposed to reflect the intensity of

---

17. See vor dem Esche, 'Die Versorgung der Bevölkerung mit Krankenhäusern', pp. 390ff.

medical care. Although the basic figures appear to be available, it is none the less difficult to make any valid judgements for the period under discussion because the way the number of hospital doctors was recorded is extremely problematic. Before the First World War, all leading senior doctors in the smaller institutions and the majority in the larger ones worked part-time. This was also true of a large number of junior doctors. It is therefore unclear what percentage of a hospital doctor's time or energy was actually devoted to caring for hospital patients and how much of it went into either scientific research (in laboratories, for example), teaching or — and this was what probably took up the most time — his private practice. From a number of nationwide surveys conducted on behalf of the Bundesrat — with all the uncertainties they entail — it is possible to calculate that in 1876, for example, there were 140,900 beds divided amongst 3,000 hospitals, with 12,000 doctors in attendance. Of these, only 334 worked exclusively in the hospitals (and even they did not regard laboratory work and teaching activities as separate from ward supervision), which meant that one 'hospital doctor' was responsible for about 422 beds. By 1898–1900 the overall situation had improved but was still far from ideal: there were 6,300 hospitals containing 370,000 beds that were supervised by 21,000 doctors. Of these, 1,927 were attached to the hospitals full-time, which meant that each 'hospital doctor' was responsible for 192 beds. By the turn of the century the intensity of medical supervision had increased, from which, even if the numerical uncertainties are taken into account, it is possible to infer that the quality of treatment available to hospital patients had also improved. At the same time — around 1900 — hospitals employed a total of 41,679 nursing staff, a ratio of one for every nine beds. These figures undoubtedly give a more accurate picture of the actual intensity of medical supervision provided in the hospitals, though it should be added that there is even considerable doubt about the reliability of the precise figures for nursing staff.[18]

However, the improvements in the quality of hospital treatment should not be measured from the increase in the intensity of medical supervision alone. In the latter years of the nineteenth and the early years of the twentieth centuries, developments in hospital care were closely bound up with the great progress made by medical science — such as improvements and refinements in examina-

18. From H. Goerke, 'Personelle und arbeitstechnische Gegebenheiten im Krankenhaus des 19. Jahrhunderts' in H. Schadewaldt (ed.), *Studien zur Krankenhausgeschichte im 19. Jahrhundert im Hinblick auf die Entwicklung in Deutschland* (Göttingen, 1976), pp. 62–6.

Determinants of the Decline in Mortality

tion techniques (the introduction of X-rays and serodiagnosis, for example), more sophisticated knowledge in the area of pathology and the discovery of whole new branches of science (for example, bacteriology and the introduction of asepsis and antisepsis in hospital treatment, especially in surgery).[19] However, advances in diagnosis and therapy, not to mention the improvements to apparatus and equipment, are more difficult to quantify and thus cannot be described on a highly aggregated level. We shall therefore have to exclude them from this present study — though of course they would provide a fertile area for further research.

In view of the difficulty of establishing reliable and unambiguous indicators that shed light on the changes in the quality of the health sector, I have in the following selected an indicator that has been tailored to fit the specific situation that existed in the period under investigation: the relationship between expenditure by disability insurance funds (*Invalidenversicherung*) on the treatment of tuberculosis and the degree of therapeutic success it achieved. The only medical measure introduced at this time which was specifically designed to check the spread of pulmonary TB among sizeable sections of the working classes in the German Empire was the treatment of relatively poor TB sufferers in public sanatoria specialising in lung diseases. This type of treatment was controversial and remains so, but it had been propagated from the mid-1890s onwards, and then quickly grew in popularity. As a result, there is a large amount of reliable data available for analysis. After 1897 this method of treating TB patients, which was prescribed when it was recognised that the individual risked being made unfit for employment, began to be financed to an increasing degree by disability insurance funds. The amount these companies spent on TB treatment rose from 107,000 Marks per year in 1893 to over 1 million Marks in 1897, over 5 million in 1901, more than 16 million in 1909 and around 18 million in 1913.[20] The number of patients who

---

19. See Aschenborn, 'Ärzte', p. 353; Goerke, 'Personelle Gegebenheiten', pp. 69ff; J.H. Wolf, 'Ausstattung und Einrichtung des Krankenhauses in Deutschland 1870–1900' in H. Schadewaldt, *Studien zur Krankenhausgeschichte*, pp. 38–55. Only hospitals could provide the environment suitable for significant progress in the realms of medical diagnosis and treatment to be made, because the equipment necessary was rarely on hand in private practices and never available to the average doctor making a house call. This is regarded as the main reason why the interest shown by bourgeois circles in hospital treatment grew rapidly from the end of the nineteenth century onwards.

20. A. Grotjahn and J. Kaup (eds), *Handwörterbuch der Sozialen Hygiene* (Leipzig, 1912), vol. 1, p. 496; *Amtliche Nachrichten des Reichs-Versicherungsamts*, Supplement 2 (1909), pp. 10–11; C. Jaenicke, 'Landesversicherungsanstalten und Tuberkulosebekämpfung, mit besonderer Berücksichtigung der Tätigkeit der Landesversicherungsanstalt Thüringen' in Blümel, *Handbuch der Tuberkulose-Fürsorge*, vol. 1, p. 181.

benefited from this funding rose from 3,334 in 1897 to 47,021 in 1913. In themselves these figures are evidence that both the resources spent and the number of those who benefited from them multiplied many times within a relatively short period of time. First and foremost, these figures record the urgency with which the fight against pulmonary TB was fought.

As far as the quality of the services provided is concerned, the figures on 'successful cures' published in the official statistical records are of greater interest.[21] Data for the period from 1897 to 1913 assembled from the statistics recorded by the Imperial Statistical Office show that, in 1897, 68 per cent of 3,334 cases had been 'successfully cured' when they were discharged from hospital. It must be said, though, that 73 per cent of those 'cured' underwent further treatment within the five-year observation period which followed their hospital stay. By 1903 the number of patients had increased by 600 per cent (20, 148). Of these as many as 80 per cent were 'cured' and the percentage of relapses had fallen to 55 per cent. Finally, in 1913, the success rate had reached an extraordinary 92 per cent, despite the fact that the number of patients had increased by over 100 per cent since 1903. The last set of figures for the number of relapses (in 1908) showed that these had fallen to 39 per cent. This seems to be evidence that the sanatorium system achieved a relative (in terms of the rather problematic notion of what actually constituted a 'cure') but appreciable degree of success. It also suggests that resources had been spent sensibly, and reflects an overall improvement in the quality of health care in what was, at the time, an extremely important area. However, it was exactly this last aspect — its social relevance — that appeared to many contemporary observers to be worth regarding as problematic. For the fact was that in the years immediately preceding the First World War, it was calculated that there were between 600,000 and 1,000,000 people suffering from pulmonary TB in the German Empire. Thus, the number of patients mentioned above who actually received treatment and on whom 16–18 million Marks were spent each year represented a maximum of 8 per cent, but probably only 5 per cent, of all those needing treatment.[22]

21. The term 'cured', which was subject to sharp criticism, implied that the patient would not have to retire within the next five years on the ground of being unfit for work. This 'success' was monitored by check-ups conducted within the five-year period. For a critique of this see Prinzing, *Handbuch*, 2nd edn, pp. 478ff.

22. In this context Grotjahn, *Soziale Pathologie*, pp. 76–93, maintains that available resources were badly invested. For an account of how the 'patient material' was pre-selected more stringently in an effort to improve the relative success of treatment, see *inter alia* H. Flatten, 'Die Bekämpfung der einzelnen übertragbaren Krankheiten' in Abel, *Handbuch der praktischen Hygiene*, vol. 1, pp. 695–6.

Determinants of the Decline in Mortality

The few available indicators that measure the changes in the quality of the health sector show quite clearly not only that there was a marked expansion of facilities during the period under discussion, but also that their quality improved noticeably. A further striking improvement concerned efficiency, especially in the hospitals, though of course the qualitative aspect of the way treatment was administered on the wards is extremely difficult to assess. One aspect of the information on the health sector that is rarely specified is the precise number of people who were able to benefit from it. The figures for the treatment of TB that were cited above demonstrate that of all those who needed some form of treatment, only a small fraction actually received it. However, to return to our principal concern with the effects of the health sector on extending average life-expectancy or reducing the mortality rate, these last statistics are also interesting from a chronological point of view. Can they be used, in view of the time to which they refer, to explain the fall in the number of deaths caused by tuberculosis?

3.3 The Relationship between the Expansion of the Health Sector and the Decline in Mortality

A consideration of these questions in relation to deaths from tuberculosis provides us with an example of how the more general theme under investigation in this chapter may be tackled. It also allows us to anticipate the conclusions drawn below in Chapter 6. Contemporary observers at the beginning of the century tended to conduct this debate from three different perspectives. The advocates of a bacteriological approach ascribed the long-term fall in TB mortality to the discovery of the tuberculosis bacillus by Robert Koch in 1882, and to the ensuing developments in the field of pharmacology. Those in favour of treatment in sanatoria felt that the fall was the direct consequence of the amount of money spent in this area, the numbers of patients treated and the success of that treatment. Thirdly, the advocates of public health measures drew attention to the efforts being made to improve sanitation and the general standard of public health.

All three arguments are put into perspective, however, by the single fact that the TB mortality rate may well have already been on the decline since the late 1820s. The debate in Germany has paid scant regard to this. A long-term survey of the city of Hamburg reveals that the TB mortality rate reached its peak in 1829; this was then followed, after a period during which it stagnated at a rather lower level, by a second rise in 1842. After that, the TB mortality rate in Hamburg began to fall (except during the war period between 1866 and 1871) and this trend continued right up to 1914. (According to the same statistics, typhus began to show a downward trend after 1842 and whooping cough after the early 1870s.[23]

Considering the relatively limited number of people who were able to benefit from treatment in a sanatorium and the fact that such treatment did not begin to be accessible to larger sections of the population until the late 1890s, it is clear that the existence of these TB sanatoria could not have affected the fall in the TB mortality rate at all before the turn of the century, and after that only in conjunction with a number of other factors.

Not even those who point to the advances of bacteriology seem to present particularly convincing arguments. Although one should guard against making generalisations on the basis of the figures for Hamburg alone, one of the conclusions that may be drawn from the statistics on Prussia discussed above is that, as a cause of death, TB was on the decline from the end of the 1870s at the latest — that is, even before the discovery of the tuberculosis bacillus. Moreover, despite Koch's discovery, there was still no effective antidote by the end of the period under discussion. The information gained about the TB germ and the way it spread, together with the development of tuberculin as an effective instrument of diagnosis, were insufficient in themselves to check the TB mortality rate. All this acquired significance only in the context of general social hygiene and public health measures. Methods of combatting sickness and disease (such as by insolating the sick, reducing the vulnerability of infection of potential sufferers by providing appropriate clothing and food, and raising the general level of domestic hygiene) which had been propagated, in part at least, since the eighteenth century without any knowledge of the bacteriological causes,[24] could now be explained more convincingly, made more

---

23. Proponents of the bacteriology thesis include Kayserling, 'Die Tuberkulose', pp. 5–6, who mentions the introduction of statutory insurance as another factor. H. Gebhard, for example, argues that treatment in medical institutions improved: 'Die Erfolge der Heilstätten für Lungenkranke' in Fränkel, *Der Stand der Tuberkulose-Bekämpfung*, pp. 159–211. For a balanced point of view from a hygienist see Prinzing, *Handbuch*, 2nd edn, pp. 474, 513–14. See also the mortality rates cited in this literature. Figures for Hamburg are taken from *Die Gesundheitsverhältnisse Hamburgs im neunzehnten Jahrhundert. Den ärztlichen Theilnehmern der 73. Versammlung Deutscher Naturforscher und Ärzte gewidmet von dem Medicinal-Collegium* (Hamburg, 1901), pp. 187, 240, 284.

24. See E.H. Ackerknecht, 'Anticontagionism between 1821 and 1867', *Bulletin of the History of Medicine*, 22 (1948).

comprehensive, and improved in specific ways. Thus Rott wrote in 1929 that the direction in which TB therapy had been progressing was only gradually altered by Robert Koch's discovery. Until well into the 1920s it largely consisted of a 'preventative form of supervision of housing conditions and economic welfare rather than of any specific form of medical care . . . In the old days, tuberculosis tended to be treated mainly by teaching and enlightening people about the importance of hygiene'.[25] However, in view of the alarming exacerbation of the housing shortage, especially in towns and cities, and the minimal amount of progress made by public and private organisations towards more effective forms of housing welfare before the First World War, the actual practical impact of educating the public on how effective hygiene was in reducing the TB mortality rate must have been very small — at least before 1900 and probably even up to 1914. Of course, in the long term, greater awareness of the problem was undoubtedly important, but it cannot be seriously regarded as the prime cause of the nationwide decline in the TB mortality rate — either alone or in combination with the treatment that people underwent in sanatoria.[26]

Since efforts to improve sanitation — to which we will return below — only marginally influenced the spread and control of tuberculosis, an explanation will have to be sought elsewhere. However, before I pursue this new line of argument, it might be advisable to re-examine changes in the configuration of the various causes of death, since this might lead us to judge the expansion of the health sector differently.

If the other major fatal diseases prevalent in the nineteenth century are included in this analysis, it is also worth noting that they began to decline at different times. The number of deaths caused by pulmonary TB, together with typhoid, began to show a basically downward trend from the end of the 1870s onwards and, as the Hamburg example demonstrated, perhaps even earlier, whilst scarlet fever began to become less prevalent in the 1880s. The mortality rate for acute infections of the respiratory organs, diphtheria and croup fell substantially for a time during the 1880s, but then rose again in an apparently cyclical fashion in the 1890s. The number of deaths caused by these diseases did not exhibit an overall downward trend until the mid-1890s. By contrast, fatalities caused by other diseases began to decline by 1887 at the latest. In

25. Rott, 'Der Rückgang', p. 98.
26. For a more recent account, which cites the various possible factors affecting TB mortality without assigning to them any particular order or significance, see Reuter, 'Verteilungs und Umverteilungseffekte', p. 145.

this context it seems important to note that the only disease that can be said to have declined as a direct result of bacteriology and therapeutic medicine was diphtheria. In the case of that disease, the mortality rate exhibited a long-term downward trend from 1895 onwards. The discovery of the diphtheria germ by Löffler, in 1883, was followed by the development of an effective serum which, after the 1890s, was soon being used extensively for the treatment of diphtheria and for vaccinations.[27] In no other instance is it possible to ascribe the progress made in combating a fatal disease exclusively to the development of medicaments or to any other direct form of medical therapy. Particularly in the case of chronic or acute infectious diseases which had been on the retreat since the early to mid-1880s, explanations must be sought outside the realms of curative medicine.

This conclusion may appear to be rather hasty because it seems to play down the improvements in diagnostic techniques (which were possible on the basis of bacteriology), on the one hand, and, on the other, the factors that contributed to more efficient medical care in hospitals. Such objections are, however, entirely theoretical and, in fact, can be shown to be unfounded. As far as the first argument is concerned, the available literature on the history of medicine contains a wealth of examples of the considerable delays that occurred before new discoveries in research were transformed into forms of therapy benefiting large numbers of people, in the form of new medicines or therapeutic techniques. It is therefore extremely misleading when medical historians attempt to portray major advances in medical treatment on the basis of a chronological survey of discoveries in medical research, dates of legislation on medicine and public health, or dates when various health-care institutions were founded.

The following few examples will serve to support this thesis. Even as late as the 1890s, not one state in the German Empire had implemented adequate measures — such as the establishment of laboratories or food research institutes — in order to guarantee the 'supervision of trade in food and luxury foodstuffs', a condition which had been prescribed in the Imperial Food Act (*Reichsnahrungsgesetz*) of 1879. It was not until after an appropriate decree had been passed by the Bundesrat in 1894 that steps were taken to found a series of institutions of this kind, and thus to guarantee a long-term if not short-term food hygiene policy. In other words, there

---

27. See Flatten, 'Die Bekämpfung', p. 748; A. Gärtner, *Leitfaden der Hygiene* (Jena, 1909), 5th edn, pp. 545–6.

was a delay of between 15 and 25 years before the law could be put into practice.[28]

An even more convincing example is provided by the campaign against acute infectious diseases — in this particular case, typhoid. Although research into a wide range of different micro-organisms as causes of sickness had been conducted since the late 1870s, effective protection against epidemics such as cholera, typhoid and others, was hampered by a shortage not only of medicine but also of the practical equipment and research institutes capable of conducting research into health and hygiene. After 1896–7, the Prussian authorities attempted to establish at least one public health laboratory in every province, which would be capable of instituting the necessary controls, conducting investigations, and so on. But these attempts were initially blocked by the presidents of the administrative districts. It was not until Robert Koch began his 'campaign against typhoid' (*Feldzug gegen den Abdominal-Typhus*) in South-West Germany at the beginning of the twentieth century, with its wide range of practical and scientific conclusions, that the final, decisive impetus was given to the foundation of a whole network of research institutes. Initially, they were located in the South-West of Prussia, though later on — largely due to Prussia's military interests — they were extended to the whole of Prussia. After 1905 all administrative districts were provided with at least one public health laboratory that was in some cases attached to a local university. It was only after this date that it became possible to speak of a systematic attempt to diagnose and combat typhoid.

Let us cite one final example. Ever since the earliest advances in bacteriological research, it had been widely appreciated that, in addition to isolating those known to be suffering from an infectious disease (a procedure that was seriously hampered by the frequent lack of reliable diagnosis), priority also had to be given to disinfecting the housing, bedding and clothing of patients. In the report on the state of health in Prussia in 1901, the existing practice on such occasions was described as follows:

> In many places — and especially in the rural areas — the possibilities of disinfection were extremely unsatisfactory right up to the end of the period covered by this report. There were shortages both of trained personnel and suitable equipment, with the result that in the vast majority of cases of infectious disease, disinfection did not take place at

---

28. On this and what follows, see D. Tutzke, 'Der Einfluss der Hygiene und Bakteriologie auf die Medizinalverwaltung in Deutschland vor 1945', *Zeitschrift für die gesamte Hygiene*, 23 (1977), pp. 868ff.

all. Where it did occur, it was often ineffective in view of the absence of expert supervision and control.[29]

Moreover, the report goes on to document the antipathy, or, at best, apathy of the vast majority of the population towards the need for disinfection, which was, after all, a vital aspect of the campaign against epidemics. For this reason, the report draws attention to the advantages to be gained from involving Catholic or Protestant nurses more closely in disinfection, presumably as a way of making it more popular.

At this point — and indeed elsewhere — in these health reports it becomes clear that, quite apart from the difficulties encountered on the scientific side (in translating scientific discoveries into some form of therapy, for example) and the possibility of delays in reacting on the part of the state legislature, it was primarily the attitudes and traditional behaviour of the population as a whole that must be held responsible for the length of time it took for certain medical innovations to become widely available. However, it should be emphasised that such negative attitudes were not found among the 'broad masses' alone. They were also prevalent in such a clearly defined group as doctors themselves. The Prussian Health Report of 1911 draws attention to the fact that the thirty-six Bacteriological Research Institutes and University Institutes of Hygiene established by that time were sufficient to cater for the needs of all the administrative districts. Doctors made use of these institutions more and more frequently as they were needed (i.e. when there were outbreaks of infectious diseases), it is claimed. They also fulfilled their obligation to report certain especially dangerous epidemics to the health authorities more frequently than they had done the previous year. None the less, the report still concludes that 'the level of demand made on the research institutes is still well short of the required target, if the campaign against epidemics is to be successful'.[30] This claim is indeed all the more understandable in view of the fact that, even in the sphere of

29. *Das Gesundheitswesen des Preußischen Staates im Jahre 1901*, p. 492.
30. *Das Gesundheitswesen des Preußischen Staates im Jahre 1911*, pp. 27ff. The following statement appeared in 1913 concerning the statutory obligation for certain infectious diseases which represented a threat to the community to be reported to the authorities: 'Apart from a very few exceptions, doctors are more willing to recognise that the legislation concerning epidemics is having entirely beneficial effects. It is a much more frequent complaint that . . . the public is less disposed to assist in these matters. The reasons for this unsatisfactory state of affairs lie in the lack of understanding of the situation, but also in indolence and a fear of inconvenience and financial cost.' From *Das Gesundheitswesen des Preußischen Staates im Jahre 1913* (Berlin, 1915), p. 19.

medical science, advances in bacteriological research, and the conclusions that could be drawn from them, were by no means universally recognised by the end of the nineteenth century, with scientists having to fight for recognition against a number of competing theories.[31]

Any objection to the assertion that therapeutic medicine was relatively ineffective in tackling the infectious diseases during the period under discussion, claiming that at least improvements in diagnostic methods would have made it possible to create more effective public health standards, must therefore be qualified. As far as everyday practice was concerned, it took several decades before the skills, instruments and institutions that had been available for use in diagnosis since the 1880s had spread to such an extent that it can be assumed that large sections of the population benefited from them. In fact, as far as the average population in the Empire was concerned, this stage does not seem to have been reached until the first decade of the twentieth century (though there was still great variation between regions and also between states).

An equal degree of scepticism is called for in the case of the other objection mentioned above, which referred to improvements in hospitals. There is no doubt that hospitals made some contribution towards checking the spread of infectious diseases, especially by isolating those infected from their social environment. It is equally true that the chances those infected had of actually surviving and convalescing may well have risen as a result of hospital treatment — especially after the introduction from the 1880s onwards of hospital wards specialising in infectious diseases. One must, however, also bear in mind that the average number of hospital beds available, particularly in rural areas, was so low as to make it highly unlikely for hospitals to be able to cope with the challenge posed by infections. In Prussia in 1913, for example, there were 42.5 beds available in general hospitals for every 10,000 inhabitants.[32] Moreover, the rather startling regional variations in medical services must be taken into consideration.

31. The vehement and prolonged nature of the dispute between advocates of the 'contagion' and the 'anti-contagion' theories, which also involved differences over fundamental political and economic convictions, is illustrated by the action of the first German Professor of Hygiene, Pettenkofer, who in 1892 drank a beakerful of a culture of cholera in order to prove that living germs could not be the cause of the disease. Like others before him, who had conducted experiments on themselves using the most varied germs, he survived. See Ackerknecht, 'Anticontagionism', pp. 567–8. For a differentiated account of competing schools of medical thought, and for criticism of Ackerknecht, see M. Pelling, *Cholera, Fever and English Medicine 1825–1865* (Oxford, 1978).

32. Calculated from *Das Gesundheitswesen des Preußischen Staates im Jahre 1913*, Appendix, pp. 2, 46; *Preußische Statistik*, vol. 90 (Berlin, 1889), p. xi, and vol. 91, p. v.

In Table 21 I have compared and contrasted the ratios of those in hospital care with the total number of deaths (including those outside hospital) for every 10,000 inhabitants of the various Prussian administrative districts in the years 1880 and 1913. The figures reveal that the degree of regional variation in the levels of hospital care was greater than the variation in the mortality rates, though by 1913 the former had become less extreme.[33] However, any reduction in regional inequality in the area of hospital care was not reflected in the mortality rates. By summarising the information given in Table 21 on this matter it is possible to deduce for 1913 the following types of relationship between the mortality rates and the percentage of people receiving hospital treatment:

(1) In Stralsund, Breslau, Münster and Aachen (i.e. 4 out of 37), both the mortality rate and the percentage of those receiving hospital treatment were higher than the Prussian average.
(2) In Berlin, Hanover, Hildesheim, Osnabrück, Arnsberg, Wiesbaden, Koblenz, Düsseldorf, Cologne and Trier (i.e. 10 out of 37), the mortality rate was lower than the Prussian average and the number of those receiving hospital care was higher.
(3) In Königsberg, Gumbinnen, Allenstein, Danzig, Marienwerder, Frankfurt an der Oder, Stettin, Köslin, Posen, Bromberg, Liegnitz, Oppeln, Magdeburg and Sigmaringen (i.e. 14 out of 37), the mortality rate was higher than the Prussian average and the percentage of those in hospital care was lower.
(4) In Potsdam, Merseburg, Erfurt, Schleswig, Lüneburg, Stade, Aurich, Minden and Kassel (i.e. 9 out of 37), both the mortality rate and the percentage of people receiving hospital treatment were lower than the Prussian average.

The most obvious hypothesis, namely that the proportion of those receiving hospital treatment is inversely proportional to the overall mortality rate is that expressed in relationship (2). This was the case in 10 out of the 37 administrative districts. It is also confirmed by the third relationship, which accounts for a further 14 districts. A total of 24 out of 37 districts (65 per cent) would seem to have conformed to this pattern. But there are also some noticeable exceptions. Despite the below-average percentage of those receiving hospital care, the mortality rates in nine of the administrative districts were also below average, and in four other cases

---

33. The variation coefficient of hospital care (as a measure of inequality) fell from 68 per cent in 1880 to 44 per cent in 1913. The corresponding figures for mortality are 11 per cent and 14 per cent.

the mortality rates were higher, despite the fact that the percentage of those in hospital care was also higher. The conclusion must therefore be that the link between the mortality rate and the percentage of those receiving hospital care can only have been indirect, and only had a *tendential* significance. An additional factor was the antipathy towards hospital shown by large sections of the population, which gradually waned, though not before the turn of the century. This was then encouraged not only by achievements in medical science but also — probably most importantly — by the establishment of statutory sickness insurance, which will be discussed in greater detail in Chapter 11 below.

Consequently, for a number of reasons, it may be assumed that during the period under investigation, the vast majority of the population of the German Empire did not, or even could not, receive hospital treatment if they contracted a contagious disease. For this reason, it is not surprising that not until the years immediately preceding the First World War did the official Prussian Health Reports began to state unequivocally that hospitals were evidently beginning to make an effective contribution to the fight against epidemics (mention was also made of the growing popularity of hospitals as institutions, and of the increasingly common opinion that those who had contracted an infectious disease should be treated in hospital).

As a final argument against the objections we have been discussing here, we can refer once again to the above discussion of the growing disparity between the different social groups with regard to the health sector, in particular with regard to the reflection of the social structure in the mortality figures. For although it is not possible to establish with any degree of certainty that the percentage of those who fell ill or even died was much higher in the working-class as a whole or even just in large sections of the lower classes, it must nevertheless be assumed that the level of social inequality in the face of death (and probably also of health) was more likely to have increased than decreased in the course of the period under discussion (we should also remember that this must be seen against the background of a general fall in the mortality rates). If, moreover, institutions such as hospitals — which were only gradually able to overcome their reputation as poorhouses and were patronised predominantly by the poorer sections of the population before 1900 — expanded in a manner as impressive as the figures indicate, and still did not manage to make a significant contribution to the establishment of more equal opportunity, then the only possible conclusion is that they were scarcely effective in tackling acute and chronic infectious diseases.

Having said all this, there is no denying that the expanding health sector did make a certain contribution towards reducing the cases of infectious disease, and thus towards the fall in the mortality rates, particularly by increasing the amount of personnel (including doctors) and hospital beds available. However, this contribution can only have been relatively small. In broaching the central question of this chapter, the arguments most worthy of consideration would seem to be those that refer to more general infrastructural improvements (especially in urban sanitation), measures to raise standards of public hygiene, improvements in the average real wage and/or the quality of diets. These arguments will be pursued in greater detail in the following chapters.

4
The Expansion of the Health-Related Infrastructure

The term 'health-related infrastructure' refers to all those institutions and, in particular, elements of the material social infrastructure which, given the criteria outlined above, cannot be included in the health sector in the strict sense of the term, but which nevertheless fulfilled a demonstrable function in terms of the rise in the standards of public hygiene that had been systematically brought about throughout the German Empire from the 1860s and 1870s onwards. With the benefit of hindsight, it can be said that the state of medical science as it existed around the middle of the nineteenth century, especially with regard to the identification of the causes of infectious diseases, the spread of infections and thus the possibility of combating such diseases, was still somewhat primitive and, in many respects, defective. Precise knowledge of the various types of infectious germ was simply unavailable, and was not even something that the majority of doctors were primarily interested in. Most of them remained convinced for several decades that infectious diseases (and especially widespread epidemics) were transmitted by poisonous vapours (or miasmas). They referred rather vaguely to the 'germs of disease', which acquired their specific qualities outside the human body, were able to survive in all sorts of dirt and from there were transmitted by humans, and by and with dirt and evil-smelling gases and vapours in particular.[34]

Although these ideas were rather vague and, partially at least, misguided when seen from a more modern perspective, they none the less formed a suitable springboard for a series of infrastructural innovations and measures to improve public hygiene, the aims of which were later acknowledged and pursued much further after discoveries in the field of bacteriology were made in the late nineteenth and early twentieth centuries. According to the 'soil or

---

34. For an account from the early part of the period under investigation see H. Eulenberg (ed.), *Handbuch des öffentlichen Gesundheitswesens* (Berlin, 1881), vol. 1, pp. 16ff.; see also Ackerknecht, 'Anticontagionism', p. 568. On public health measures see Eulenberg, pp. 376–81, 556ff.

ground theory' (*Boden-oder Platz-Theorie*) developed by Pettenkofer, the first German professor of hygiene, the epidemics that commanded most attention (the plague, cholera, yellow fever) could be effectively controlled by keeping the subsoil as pure as possible, preventing the processes of decay and the formation of gases and simultaneously strengthening the human body's immunity to infection. A number of specific measures to improve hygiene were introduced, and consisted of isolating the sick (though the authorities had practised quarantine as a method of controlling the bubonic plague ever since the Middle Ages), cleaning houses and streets, encouraging the use of disinfectants, preserving the purity of drinking-water and encouraging a healthier diet and life style. The doctors' role in this was restricted to diagnosis, on the one hand, and to imposing quarantine and providing disinfectants, on the other, together with writing and distributing information designed to educated people about healthier diets and life styles. However, the number of people who responded to doctors' involvement of this kind must have been extremely small until well into the 1880s and was limited to the small number of patients who actually consulted a doctor, or to the occasions when doctors who looked after the poor, or district medical officers, recognised the danger of epidemics whilst on their rounds. Diagnoses and suggestions put forward by doctors and public health specialists could only lead to greater efficiency in the campaign to prevent or cure cases of infection if they were taken up and put into practice by the state authorities (in the form of compulsory quarantine, for example). However, with the exception of the campaign against smallpox, which had succeeded with the help of the smallpox vaccine administered consistently in some German states since the early nineteenth century, for a long time the authorities generally reacted too late, with inadequate resources and on too small a scale. Since the miasma theory of infectious germs blamed high levels of sickness on gases and vapours released by processes of decay and fermentation, disinfection that was intended to check the spread of epidemics was often restricted to eliminating various evil smells and the sources thereof.

However, in the wake of a series of new measures introduced by the authorities with the specific intention of improving public health and hygiene, reductions were achieved in the long term in the numbers and effects of epidemics, together with improvements in the overall level of health and a decline in the mortality rates. From the middle of the nineteenth century onwards, these measures had been initiated by various public health specialists, and were then taken up and put into practice by a number of local governments. At the time they were summarised in the expression 'urban sanitation' (*Städte-Assanierung*). The result was a whole series of decisive infrastructural improvements to the urban environment with regard to the drinking-water supply, sewerage and refuse disposal, street-cleaning and domestic hygiene. This period witnessed the development of municipal water works, especially in the towns (with increasingly effective filter processes), extensive drainage systems, municipal refuse disposal, street-cleaning and — after a considerable delay — housing welfare. Since the first steps to establish the latter were not really taken until the 1890s, and even then took some considerable time before having any widespread impact, and since refuse disposal and street-cleaning were regarded as being of secondary importance in eliminating infectious diseases, we must focus our attention at this point on the drinking water supply and sewage disposal systems and on their effect on the changes we have discussed in the general level of the 'people's health'. The question remains, however, whether supplying an increasing percentage of the population with purified drinking water, and hygienically disposing of sewage, including faeces, by means of a central drainage system really can be shown to have had a direct effect on the reduction in the average mortality rates, and if so, from which point in time.

4.1 Drinking-water Supplies and Sewerage Systems

In the following attempt to arrive at some initial answers to these questions, it will be assumed that washing- and drinking-water which is heavily polluted and riddled with germs represents a considerable threat to health. It can facilitate the transmission of infectious diseases (especially large-scale epidemics) and skin disease, not to mention all sorts of other bacteria that may upset the metabolism or be detrimental to health in some other way. In view of this, the washing- and drinking-water supplied to the German population must be judged to have been extremely inadequate until the late nineteenth and early twentieth centuries. The state of affairs in 1900 can be illustrated by citing some figures taken from a private survey of water supplies in the German Empire (see Table 22). This shows that of the 972 Prussian towns with more than 2000 inhabitants in 1895, 42 per cent operated a central water supply system. It also shows, however, that the inhabitants of 58 per cent of towns were dependent on wells, water tanks or natural water supplies for their drinking- and washing-water. Of the 892 Prussian rural communities of this size, no more than 20 per cent had some form of central water supply, which means, of course, that the inhabitants of 80 per cent of these communities continued to obtain their water from traditional sources.

Perhaps even these figures paint too rosy a picture. A breakdown of Prussian towns into different sizes reveals that, in 1895, 81 per cent of towns with a population of more than 10,000 possessed a modern water supply, while this was true of only 49 per cent of towns with between 5,000 and 10,000 inhabitants, 28 per cent of towns with 3,000 and 5,000 and, finally, 16 per cent of towns with between 2,000 and 3,000 (see Table 22). It should also be remembered that the two smallest categories alone covered 55 per cent of all towns with more than 2,000 inhabitants. The ratios for the whole of the German Empire are slightly better, but they also reflect the same tendency for the quality of the water supply to deteriorate the smaller the community. It must be concluded, then, that 30 per cent — at the very most — of villages and rural communities outside Prussia with less than 2,000 inhabitants, and a maximum of 16 per cent in Prussia, were served by some form of central water supply. (The criterion here is the extent to which towns with 2,000 to 3,000 inhabitants had such systems.)

Unfortunately, these figures refer to the towns rather than the inhabitants themselves. However, to emphasise the importance of the remarks just made on the numbers of communities without a central water supply, it should be remembered that in 1900 46 per cent of the total population of the German Empire still lived in towns or villages with less than 2,000 inhabitants. As far as Prussia itself is concerned, more reliable figures are available from surveys conducted on behalf of the presidents of the administrative districts. As a result it is possible to estimate with a reasonable degree of accuracy what percentage of the inhabitants of the individual administrative districts had access to water supplied from a modern, central water works (see Table 23). What is immediately conspicuous is the extreme degree of regional variation and the clear disparities between the more heavily populated and industrialised regions, on the one hand, and the predominantly agricultural areas, on the other. The proportions of people whose water came from a central supply system were lowest in a few Eastern districts (between 5 and 20 per cent). Even as late as 1900, an average of over 60 per cent of the Prussian population depended on wells and water tanks for its water supply. Thanks to the greater efforts made in a few states in the South, the percentage of the non-Prussian popula-

Determinants of the Decline in Mortality

tion of the Empire whose water was supplied from a central works was probably somewhat higher, though it must be assumed that even outside Prussia no more than half the population had access to an up-to-date water system. To this extent then, much-quoted statistics published by the Imperial Health Office in 1903 are grossly misleading in that they claim that only a little over 4 per cent of the populations of towns with 15,000 or more inhabitants were not 'connected' to the central water supply.[35] This extremely favourable figure fails to take account of the fact that only about 32 per cent of the total population actually lived in towns of this size, and that the smaller the community, the less likely it was to have a central waterworks. Thus, the survey conducted by the Imperial Health Office does not contain any reliable information on the average percentage of the total population that was supplied from a central water system and, on the contrary, must be qualified in view of the vast disparities between town and country and the different sizes of towns and villages.

We scarcely need to reiterate that the importance of a central water supply system with efficient filtering, for it is clear that human — and industrial — waste were the major sources of pollution in drinking- and washing-water which were dangerous to human health. The urgent need for central water supply systems would undoubtedly have been reduced if drainage had been systematically installed in towns and villages, and sewage had been channelled so that it did not seep into the surface or ground water used for drinking or washing. Quite apart from the fact that many of the sewerage schemes that were begun during the period under discussion were by no means guarantees against pollution of surface and ground water (because the sewage was released into natural waterways in a semi- or completely unpurified state), the following figures are evidence of the extremely slow rate at which sewerage systems were built throughout Germany. After the first sewerage schemes were completed in a few towns in the 1850s, little effort was made in the following twenty years to expand them. Instead there were a number of heated and, from a socio-historical perspective, extremely interesting, debates in a large number of local councils (who would commission construction work) between those in favour of a sewerage system and those against.[36] Usually it was those in favour who won in the end, but it

---

35. See *Statistisches Jahrbuch für das Deutsche Reich*, vol. 26 (1905), p. 301.
36. See P.R. Gleichmann, 'Die Verhäuslichung körperlicher Verrichtungen' in idem et al. (eds), *Materialen zu Norbert Elias' Zivilisationstheorie* (Frankfurt am Main, 1979), pp. 254–78. For a more general analysis of the relationship between urbanisa-

all served considerably to delay the preliminary phases of building programmes (in the course of which lengthy reports based on sound evidence were usually presented by both sides and then debated).

In Prussia for example, in no more than twenty-six towns, with a total population of 2.7 million people, had a sewerage system been finished by 1883.[37] If this is compared with the total population of all towns of more than 2000 inhabitants (9.7 million), then it becomes clear that at this time only a little more than a quarter (27.3 per cent) lived in towns with a sewerage system. Even in such cases there was no guarantee that all or even most of the inhabitants of these towns could actually avail themselves of that system. Although the construction of sewerage systems reached a peak in Germany between 1890 and 1910, even as late as 1907 no more than 66.5 per cent of the people living in Prussian towns with more than 2000 inhabitants had access to sewerage systems. Leaving aside the cities (i.e. those communities with more than 100,000 inhabitants), the percentage of the urban population that benefited from a sewerage system was no more than 55 per cent. We see here again the same pattern of smaller communities tending to be much worse off than larger towns and cities. Even in 1907 there were still enormous disparities in sewage disposal facilities, and thus in public health standards in Prussia. This view is confirmed by the fact that only one million of the total rural population — i.e. around 5 per cent of all the inhabitants of the country areas — had access to a sewerage system. Or, to put it the other way round, 19.4 million people living in the rural districts of Prussia were without a sewerage system even as late as 1914.

---

tion, housing conditions and health, see J. Bleker, 'Die Stadt als Krankheitsfaktor. Eine Analyse ärztlicher Auffassungen im 19. Jahrhundert', *Medizinhistorisches Journal*, 18(1/2) (1983), pp. 118–36; J.-P. Goubert, 'Public Hygiene and Mortality Decline in France in the 19th Century' in T. Bengtsson et al. (eds), *Pre-industrial Population Change. The Mortality Decline and Short-term Population Movements* (Stockholm, 1984), pp. 151–9; A.L. Greer and S. Greer (eds), *Cities and Sickness. Health Care in Urban America* (Beverly Hills, 1983); B. Luckin, 'Death and Survival in the City: Approaches to the History of Disease', *Urban History Yearbook* (1980), pp. 53–62; idem, 'The Final Catastrophe — Cholera in London, 1866', *Medical History*, 21(1) (1977), pp. 32–42; G. Rosen, 'Economic and Social Policy in the Development of Public Health', in idem, *From Medical Police to Social Medicine: Essays in the History of Health Care* (New York, 1974), pp. 176–200; idem, 'Disease, Debility and Death', in H.J. Dyos and M. Wolff (eds), *The Victorian City. Images and Reality* (London and Boston, 1973), vol. 2, pp. 625–67; idem, *A History of Public Health* (New York, 1958); J. von Simson, *Kanalisation und Städtehygiene im 19. Jahrhundert* (Düsseldorf, 1983); R. Woods and J. Woodward (eds), *Urban Disease and Mortality in Nineteenth-Century England* (London and New York, 1984).

37. See Salomon, 'Beseitigung der Abwässer und Abfallstoffe. Reinhaltung der Wasserläufe' in Rapmund, *Das Preußische Medizinal- und Gesundheitswesen*, pp. 106ff.

The Prussian Health Report of 1911 remarked: 'Many houses in country villages and small towns do not have any form of privy . . . In the towns many people continue to complain about the nuisance caused by the smells produced when privies are emptied.'[38] We can see from the wealth of information and comments contained in these health reports that, towards the end of the period under examination, the installation of a well-sealed cesspool from which faeces were periodically emptied, or, after preliminary filtering, directed through a trickling filter system, was still clearly felt to provide the optimum solution, though it was one which in most cases was far from being implemented in the smaller towns and was even less common in the rural areas. Instead, throughout the first decade of the twentieth century, reports regularly came in from all Prussian administrative districts listing a wide range of grievances. In the main these complaints revolved around the fact that the wells (on which, as was shown above, the majority of those living in country areas were dependent for their water supply) were in close proximity to leaking latrines, cesspits, cowsheds and containers of sludge, and that the wells themselves had leaking walls and were not covered. The Health Report of 1901 concludes: 'This explains why reports have been received from almost all districts of epidemics of typhoid caused by infected water'.[39] The appalling state of drinking-water supplies and sewage disposal in Munich that Pettenkofer had strongly criticised during the 1850s was still commonplace 50 years later in many parts of Germany, especially in rural areas. The 'Public Health Campaign' (*Kampf der Hygieniker*) against this deplorable state of affairs was still in full cry as late as 1914.

It is no surprise that, compared with projects to construct central water supply systems, sewerage schemes were generally initiated later, took longer to complete, and by the end of the period under discussion had affected a much smaller percentage of the German population. There were probably a number of reasons: the considerably greater technical demands imposed by sewerage systems; the more extensive pressures on the population to change its everyday behaviour (linked to certain profound changes in individual and group values and in the norms of social interaction which we have not yet discussed); the sharp increase in the amount of administration (which led to the creation of new municipal administrative functions, and the institutions associated with them,

---

38. *Das Gesundheitswesen des Preußischen Staates im Jahre 1911*, p. 357.
39. *Das Gesundheitswesen des Preußischen Staates im Jahre 1901*, p. 279.

that had the power to exert a lasting influence on people's everyday lives); and, finally, the far greater sums of money involved.

In view of these factors, there was an even more urgent need to expand and develop central water supply systems, but, as we have shown above, it was not until the end of the nineteenth century a large section of the population began to receive water from such systems. Even as late as 1914, about half the total population was still excluded. Moreover, even the statistical information that is cited in this context is to a large extent rather unreliable. In the first place, the surveys usually fail to indicate the quality of the installations concerned which, in the early phases in particular (the 1860s and 1870s), tended to use surface water which had not been adequately filtered. Secondly, they also obscure the fact that a considerable amount of time usually passed before the whole population of a town or village could be connected up to the newly installed system. The statistics claim that the whole population of a town or village was provided for from the moment the first sections of the systems were opened. It need scarcely be said that a central water supply system is less able to function successfully as a form of protection against infectious diseases (especially epidemics), not to mention a host of other threats to physical welfare — in other words to contribute towards improving the overall level of health and reducing the mortality rate — unless it serves the highest possible proportion of the population, and not simply a few small isolated groups. The dates on which waterworks were installed in larger towns (i.e. those with more than 25,000 inhabitants) which, according to the statistics, were mostly — or even completely — connected to a water system from a very early date, are particularly misleading. According to the data, 54 per cent of such towns had been equipped with a modern system by 1880, 77 per cent by 1890, and an extraordinary 100 per cent by 1900 (see Table 24). Berlin was one of the cities in this category, and in the literature on the subject it is usually claimed that Berlin's water came from a central supply early as 1856.[40] However, in order to demonstrate what sort of time-scales were actually involved — at least in cities like Berlin

---

40. A work typical of many others is E. Gerlach and K. Hünerberg, *Die Wasserversorgung* (Munich and Vienna, 1963), 6th and expanded edn, p. 17; see also von Simson, Kanalisation. For an example of a socio-historical view, see R.J. Evans, 'Social Inequality in the Face of Death and Disease in 19th-Century Hamburg', paper presented to the 8th UEA Research Seminar in Modern German Social History on 'Health und Medicine', Norwich, University of East Anglia, Norwich, 9–10 January 1985 (available as duplicated manuscript); idem, 'Die Cholera und die Sozialdemokratie: Arbeiterbewegung, Bürgertum und Staat in Hamburg während der Krise von 1892' in A. Herzig et al. (eds), *Arbeiter in Hamburg* (Hamburg, 1983), pp. 203–13.

Determinants of the Decline in Mortality

— and to expose the social disparities which generally accompanied the way such infrastructural improvements were made, we shall now look in greater detail at the data available on the development of the water supply and sewerage systems in Berlin. (More universally applicable versions of the conclusion we shall draw below on Berlin would only be possible on the basis of a large number of local studies — another project for the future.)

4.2 Case Study: Berlin

It is sometimes claimed that Berlin had a central water supply system from as early as 1852. However, that year merely marks the establishment of the company that was set up to build a water works. Building commenced in 1853, and the works became operational in 1856. Its primary function was to supply water for the watering of gutters. Individual private properties could be connected to these mains but, owing to cost (and, in some cases, a 'lack of judgement on the part of the house-owners'), very few were in fact connected in the early years. A further phase of joining up private houses to the mains was completed at the beginning of the 1860s, but the total represented no more than a tiny percentage of all properties, and this situation continued until the mid-1870s. Moreover, since the system was fed with surface water taken from the River Spree above Berlin and then passed through sand filters, the quality of the water supplied left a great deal to be desired from the point of view of hygiene. In any event, plans to connect every single property to the water mains would undoubtedly have ended in failure in view of the system's limited capacity. In 1873 no more than 8,114 of the 15,047 properties (i.e. 54 per cent), which housed 50 per cent of Berliners (437,864 out of 882,460), were connected to the mains.[41] It was not until the early 1880s, and the opening of new waterworks with a vastly improved filter system, that the majority of old and new buildings located within the city boundaries were connected to the central water supply. Thus, the real extension of the water supply occured in the late 1870s and early 1880s, at least as far as properties were concerned. Of course, we should not be led to conclude that all private homes and flats were connected to the mains. That this was not the case emerges, for

---

41. Taken from *Die Anstalten der Stadt Berlin für die öffentliche Gesundheitspflege und für den naturwissenschaftlichen Unterricht. Festschrift dargeboten den Mitgliedern der 59. Versammlung Deutscher Naturforscher und Ärzte von den städtischen Behörden* (Berlin, 1886), p. 243.

example, from the 1879 amendments to the Police Regulations (*Polizeiverordnung*) and local byelaws (*Ortsstatut*) (of 1874) which stated quite clearly that a property could be regarded as connected to the mains (now these improvements were being supported by the authorities) 'if the residents of each inhabited building have access to at least one tap connected to the mains and a sink underneath it'.[42] The percentage of Berlin homes with such facilities increased as follows: 19 in 1864, 32 in 1867, 37 in 1871, 43 in 1875, 80 in 1880, 85 in 1885 and 93 in 1890.[43]

From the point of view of hygiene, the expansion of the water supply system was a resounding success. Although the standard of the supply in the late 1870s would not meet today's requirements, the impact it was having by that time is demonstrated by the fact that the incidence of death from typhoid, a disease which reacted particularly sensitively to the purification of water, fell dramatically between 1875 and 1880. Apart from a few sudden jumps in years which had seen epidemics, an average of around 10 people in every 10,000 died of typhoid each year during the 1850s. In the 1860s, the figure fell slightly to around 8.2 in every 10,000. The rate remained at over 8 from 1873 to 1875, then dropped for the first time in 1877 to 2.1 and remained at this level until the beginning of the 1880s. From 1881 to 1883 it rose again briefly to 3.6, only to fall again in 1884 to less than 2 in 1885. After 1890, the disease killed less than 1 person in 10,000.[44] During the second half of the 1870s — i.e. the period in which the proportion of homes connected to the water mains rose rapidly from just over 50 per cent to 90 per cent and over — the number of deaths caused by typhoid in Berlin fell to one-third of its 'traditional' level (that is, the average over the previous 20 years). And all this in spite of the fact that, as will be shown below, an ideal solution to the problem of sewerage had by no means been found, and the differences, in the quality of the actual water supply and sewage disposal facilities consolidated or in some cases even amplified the social inequalities between the various urban residential districts.

But let us first turn our attention to the problem of sewerage. Until well into the 1870s Berlin's sewerage system consisted of no more than a network of irrigated gutters — covered and open —

42. Ibid., p. 262.
43. From R. Böckh (ed.), *Die Bevölkerungs- und Wohnungs-Aufnahme vom 1. December 1885 in der Stadt Berlin* (Berlin, 1891), no. 2, section 4, p. 69; idem, *Die Bevölkerungs- und Wohnungs-Aufnahme vom 1. December 1890 in der Stadt Berlin* (Berlin, 1893), no. 1, section 4, p. 26.
44. See T. Weyl, 'Assanierung' in idem (ed.), *Soziale Hygiene* (Jena, 1904), p. 17 (Weyl's *Handbuch der Hygiene*, 4th supplementary volume).

Determinants of the Decline in Mortality

which simply flowed into open lakes, rivers or canals. One effect of the gradual introduction of the water closet during the 1860s was a rapid deterioration in the hygienic standard of such conduits.

It was not until the beginning of the 1870s that expert opinion became available which could be used as a basis for practical policy (Virchow's 'General Report' of 1872, and Hobrecht's plans for a new drainage system, for example). In the ensuing years, the authorities set about constructing a central sewerage system, and by the end of the 1870s many properties had been connected to it. By 1885–6, 16,251 out of 18,216 properties in Berlin (i.e. around 90 per cent) had been linked to it.[45] This seems to suggest that the vast majority of Berliners had been provided with a hygienically acceptable form of sewage disposal within the space of a decade. Although the sewerage system took longer to construct than the water supply system, in both cases the most important stages in construction took place during the late 1870s and early 1880s, with each system complementing the other in checking the spread of infectious diseases.

In more general terms, these developments helped to bring about more equal opportunities, for, despite the increased availability of a central water supply and the gradual abandonment of the simple leach-pit system of sewage disposal,[46] disparities in the facilities available to different social groups had initially grown dramatically until the mid-1870s. In Table 25, I have compared and contrasted a few of the more prosperous districts of Berlin with some of the less privileged areas, classified principally in terms of the proportion of households with servants, and of the percentage of homes which housed more than four people in each heated room. I have compared these districts in terms of the proportion of homes connected to the central water supply and equipped with WCs in the two sample years 1875 and 1890. As far as the provision of a water supply and WCs is concerned, the disparity between the richer and poorer areas actually decreased considerably between 1875 and 1890 (see Table 25, columns 6 to 9). It is therefore all the more surprising that the average mortality rates, which have also been recorded in Table 25 (columns 11 and 12) continued to vary

45. See *Die Anstalten der Stadt Berlin*, p. 262.
46. In 1875 only 4.1 per cent of developed properties in Berlin were connected to a vault system, which was the most hygienic method of waste treatment and disposal apart from sewerage systems. Even some of these also used the particularly problematic system of cesspits or trickling filters, to which 57 per cent of developed properties had access. In addition there was an unspecified number of cases where excrement flowed directly from privies into open watercourses or into gutters. See R. Böckh (ed.), *Die Bevölkerungs-, Gewerbe- und Wohnungs-Aufnahme vom 1. Dezember 1875 in der Stadt Berlin* (Berlin, 1878), no. 1, section 1, p. 94.

considerably between the more prosperous and the poorer areas, even though they fell overall in both cases.

We must bear in mind, of course, that the average level of health — and thus mortality — was affected by a whole range of different factors, of which the water supply and sewerage system were but two. It is therefore possible that infrastructural facilities were generating more equal opportunities even when mortality rates continued to vary considerably among social groups. Perhaps it would be more plausible to ascribe the overall downward trend in the mortality rates in particular to the improvements in the infrastructural facilities available to each social category as well as to the fact that the disparities between them were reduced. And yet, on closer analysis, the figures in Table 25 obscure genuine differences in the quality and quantity of facilities available to each group. Column 10 reveals, for example, that in the poorer areas, WCs were often installed in the tenement stairwell and served as communal WCs for several different flats rather than for single domestic units. Since the relative number of people per living space was higher in such areas, and in view of the fact that most WCs were communal, standards of hygiene associated with these conditions were less likely to improve in the poorer areas than in the richer ones. In fact, the installation of communal WCs serving a number of frequently overcrowded houses may well have simply created yet another source of infection. Bearing in mind that in 1890 the proportion of households without access to any sort of WC was still much higher in the poorer areas than in the more prosperous ones, and also that the alternative was the much-criticised leach-pit system (rather than the sewage — or septic-tank — system, which Virchow regarded as the lesser evil), the combination of the percentage of homes without a WC of any kind and the percentage of hygienically substandard communal WCs indicates that, in all, the poorer areas were substantially worse off. On average the proportion of housing of inferior standards of hygiene was approximately one-third higher than in the better-off areas. This situation may well have influenced the corresponding disparities in the mortality rates. We might presume that various fatal infectious diseases continued to prosper on account of lack of hygiene prevalent in some of the poorer areas long after they had been 'banished' from the wealthier parts. However, empirical evidence would suggest otherwise, particularly that relating to the incidence of typhoid between 1880 and 1895 in the areas of Berlin listed in Table 25. What is perhaps most remarkable is that, as early as 1885, the numbers of those suffering from typhoid, and especially those in the less privileged areas, fell dramatically, which resulted in a reduction in the disparities in the incidence of typhoid in the various areas. By 1895 they had almost disappeared altogether. While in 1880 there was still a clear link between the quality of the infrastructure in each area and the proportion of people suffering from typhoid (at least as far as districts of a relatively homogenous social composition were concerned), by 1895 the differences in infrastructural hygiene levels, though they persisted, no longer seemed to be reflected in the numbers of typhus cases.

These findings are similar to the evidence we found to show that the differences in mortality rates between the privileged and underprivileged urban areas were decreasing, as were those between the mortality rates in the latter and the Berlin average: all these suggest that life chances were becoming increasingly uniform. There can be little doubt that the construction of a public water supply and sewage disposal system played a direct part in bringing this about, as did the resulting widespread improvements in the standard of hygiene of the general environment. Since, however, mortality levels continued to vary from district to district, other overlapping factors bearing upon social differentiation (the 'components of market situation, or market capacity'), which had very little connection with the health-related infrastructure, have to be taken into consideration. While relative inequalities did become less marked, the effects of these factors could never be completely eliminated by the infrastructure and could only be reduced. In this respect, the dangers associated with particular types of work, the standard of housing and quality of diet, both of which were linked to income, are particularly significant, for such factors determine the degree to which an individual is exposed to infection, and his or her ability to resist it. We can provide further evidence for this by calculating some correlative values for 1875 and 1885, the years between which the Berlin water supply system was expanded to include a total of 13 registry office districts. (Figures for eight of these are shown in Table 25). In 1875, the inverse relationship between the availability of a central water supply system and the average mortality rate was extremely weak ($r = -0.47$), and by 1885 this had only slightly increased ($r = -0.63$). By contrast, the significance for mortality of 'wealth', indicated by whether servants were employed or not, would seem to have been paramount (1875, $r = -0.65$; 1885, $r = -0.94$).

4.3 Summary

We have looked here at the details of infrastructural expansion and its probable effects on the average level of public health. We should not, however, forget how little the majority of the population of the German Empire was able to profit from these developments before 1900. It should also be remembered that for the whole of the period under analysis — that is until the early years of the twentieth century — large sections of the populations of small towns and the majority of the rural population were virtually excluded from the developments we have been examining. However, even among such people the mortality rate must have fallen. Since they represented such a large percentage of the population, there could not otherwise have been such a clear fall in the national average mortality rate. Thus, whilst from the 1880s onwards the urban population (especially in medium-sized and large towns) had been benefiting from an improved health-related infrastructure, a number of other additional factors affecting the mortality rate and the rise in the average life expectancy must also be taken into consideration — especially where the rural population is concerned. In accordance with the overall theoretical framework outlined above, we should now move away from the whole question of the 'health service' and the 'health-related infrastructure' and concentrate on the improvements in the average standard of living and the quality of the average diet.

5
Changes in Income and Diet

It seems likely that improvements in the average standard of living occurred in the last third of the nineteenth century, and that this led to a rise in the overall quality of food consumed. In turn, people's capacities to resist infection were enhanced, with the result that average mortality rates fell and the general level of health rose. There may have been a great reduction in the chronic protein deficit, a consequence of mal- and undernutrition in large sections of the population during the first half of the nineteenth century in Germany, which up to the 1860s had increased the likelihood of infection in children and young people in particular. Above all, children and teenagers may have become more immune to infection since the 1870s, a fact that would correlate with the variations in the mortality rates in different age groups mentioned above. Evidence available to support our assumptions here is even more meagre than that used above, and has been even less systematically processed. All I can do here is refer to a number of different ideas, the validity of which might be a subject for future debate.

It is not my intention to enter into a general discussion of the standard of living.[47] None the less, one indisputably important piece of information that should be mentioned here is that, in real terms, the average income in Germany almost doubled in the course of the period under discussion.[48] By 1913 it was more than 60 per cent higher than the average during the whole of the 1870s. The rate of increase was reasonably constant throughout, with the exception of a few cyclical fluctuations. Of course, when seen in the light of clear regional and social variations in the levels of income and wealth, this information seems to provide a distorted picture, and should not be interpreted as a sign that standards of living in contrasting social groups were converging. Nevertheless, the index

---

47. See A. Triebel, 'Lebensstandarddebatten in der modernen Sozialgeschichtsschreibung. Ein Literaturbericht' (unpublished manuscript, University of Bielefeld, 1977); idem, 'Differential Consumption', and the literature discussed there.
48. See T.J. Orsagh, 'Löhne in Deutschland 1871–1913: Neuere Literatur und weitere Ergebnisse', *Zeitschrift für die gesamte Staatswissenschaft*, 125 (1969), p. 481.

is a faithful expression of trends in the real incomes of large sections of the population, especially in the towns. The pattern is also reinforced by other more general information. One fact that is worthy of particular attention in this context is that in the course of the first half of the period under discussion — a time when there was a marked rise in average real incomes — waged and salaried employees in the German Empire benefited from a considerable improvement in the relative distribution of income (total income per dependent income earner divided by total profit per self-employed person), compared with the situation in 1870. The ratio improved markedly during the depression of the late 1870s, fell slightly in the early 1880s but then remained at a fairly high level until the beginning of the 1890s. It was not until 1895–9 that the relative distribution of income fell below the level of the early 1870s.[49] From then on it fell steadily until the end of our period, though this was compensated to a large extent, as far as the average standard of living was concerned, by the growth in the gross national product, which had been accelerating since the mid-1890s.

It would thus appear that even large sections of the working-class population must have had the opportunity to improve their average daily diet in terms of both quality and quantity. Since the turn of the century, the trend within all sections of the working-class population had been towards stricter birth control and thus towards a reduction in the number of mouths to feed, which presumably would have helped families adopt better dietary habits in a period that was marked by a sharp increase in the cost of living. There is also a good deal of evidence that suggests that this is what actually happened. In a series of studies, Teuteberg was able to argue convincingly that the second half of the nineteenth century was not only characterised by a tangible rise in the per-capita consumption of potatoes, cereals and meat, but also that a growing proportion of the less privileged income-groups were affected.[50] In

49. See A. Jeck, *Wachstum und Verteilung des Volkseinkommens* (Tübingen, 1970), p. 100. The relative position of dependent wage-earners in the pattern of distribution is defined here as the earned income per dependent earner divided by income from profit per self-employed earner (p. 12).

50. See H.J. Teuteberg, 'Studien zur Volksernährung unter sozial- und wirtschaftsgeschichtlichen Aspekten' in idem and G. Wiegelmann, *Der Wandel der Nahrungsgewohnheiten unter dem Einfluß der Industrialisierung* (Göttingen, 1972), pp. 118–32, 156–62, 183; idem, 'Der Verzehr von Nahrungsmitteln in Deutschland pro Kopf und Jahr seit Beginn der Industrialisierung (1850–1975). Versuch einer quantitativen Langzeitanalyse', *Archiv für Sozialgeschichte*, 19 (1979), pp. 331–88; idem, 'Wie ernährten sich Arbeiter im Kaiserreich?' in Conze and Engelhardt, *Arbeiterexistenz*, pp. 57–73; idem, 'Food Consumption in Germany since the Beginning of Industrialization: A Quantitative Longitudinal Approach' in H. Baudet and H. van der Meulen (eds), *Consumer Behaviour and Economic Growth in the Modern Economy* (London and Canberra, 1982), pp. 233–77.

addition, it is possible to infer from Teuteberg's studies that the quality of composition of the average diet also improved — for example in the form of a relative decline in the amount of potatoes consumed and their replacement by cereals, especially wheat flour or bread, and an increase in meat consumption. These detailed findings complement the estimated annual calorie consumption in Germany after 1850, calculated by Hoffmann et al.[51] In their survey, Hoffmann et al. contrasted actual consumption with recommended levels of consumption, and discovered that it was not until the second half of the 1870s that these balanced out for the first time. There was a further brief slump between 1880 and 1884 (when the ratio of actual to recommended consumption was lower than it had been in the early 1870s), but from the second half of the 1880s onwards the estimated actual consumption of calories far exceeded the recommended amount. However, we should not forget that these estimates were often rather approximate, and this has exposed them to serious criticism, especially from dieticians and nutritionists.[52] While, unfortunately, we cannot claim that the figures are absolutely precise, in the context of a long-term comparison they probably give a fairly accurate indication of a genuine trend towards a rise in average annual per-capita calorie consumption.

In his detailed analysis of the reasons for the fall in the mortality rate in the Eastern provinces of Prussia in the course of the nineteenth century, Dickler has shown that the rise in the per-capita consumption of cereals, which contributed towards the improvement in the quality of the average diet, was a reflection of structural changes in the German cereals market. Long-run shifts of emphasis in the world cereals market put sustained pressure on cereal prices. Now that relatively cheap foreign cereals were beginning to find their way onto the German market in large quantities and, at the same time, domestic wheat, which had lost its traditional export markets, was being sold in increasing quantities on the home market, conditions for an increase in cereals consumption were extremely favourable — even without the rise in the average real wage. What is even more significant, however, is that Dickler was able to use the Eastern provinces of Prussia as an example to demonstrate the extremely close connection between an improvement in the quality of the average diet, and the decline in the percentage of deaths caused by acute infectious diseases.[53] This

---

51. See Hoffmann et al. *Das Wachstum*, p. 659.
52. See Teuteberg, 'Der Verzehr', pp. 385ff.
53. See Dickler, *Labour Market Pressure*, p. 186–7, 193–203.

would explain why mortality among children and young people fell even in rural Prussia — areas that were clearly underprivileged as far as medical services and the health-related infrastructure were concerned (see Tables 18 and 21).

Rises in the real average incomes of employees, and temporary improvements in their relative position in the pattern of income distribution, are generally felt to have been consequences of the accelerating process of industrialisation that had been taking place since the late 1860s and early 1870s. Workers in the growth industries, who also made up a large part of the population in industrial conurbations, would be particularly favoured. Moreover, statutory sickness insurance was initially limited to this group of workers.[54] By contrast, certain groups of unskilled workers, who found it difficult to adjust to the urban industrial life style, were excluded from this development. The majority of peasants and farm labourers found themselves in the same position. Against this background, the results of Dickler's above-mentioned study are all the more important. He convincingly demonstrates that the comparatively small, yet appreciable, increase in the ratio of doctors to the population and in the numbers of hospital beds could not really have had any noticeable effect on the fall in the proportion of deaths caused by acute and chronic infectious diseases. The same was true of improvements in the health-related infrastructure. All this makes the part played by improvements in real average incomes and the quality of the average diet even more significant.

After the turn of the century, the principal new factor affecting the average mortality rate was the onset of a downward trend in infant mortality. As I showed above, this was due primarily to a sharp fall in the proportion of deaths from gastro-intestinal infections. It is obvious that the improvements in both the health-related infrastructure and the average diet cannot have been the main reasons for this. If they had been, the effects would have been registered some ten to 20 years earlier. As was indicated above, however, infant mortality rates in all sections of the working class — i.e. in the vast majority of the population — did not really begin to decline until the turn of the century. People generally made little use of the improved medical care or of the chance to consult a doctor in an independent practice or hospital, even when these

---

54. See Tennstedt, 'Sozialgeschichte', p. 386; R. Baron makes some very astute comments about the political consequences of placing limitations on the people who were favoured in this way in 'Weder Zuckerbrot noch Peitsche. Historische Konstitutionsbedingungen des Sozialstaats in Deutschland', *Beiträge zur Marxschen Theorie* (Frankfurt am Main, 1979), vol. 12, pp. 40–8.

facilities were well within the geographical and financial reach of those concerned. Instead, we can assume that, together with the effects of the falling birth rate after 1900 (a further reason for the fall in the infant mortality rate), there were primarily two significant additional factors. In many regions of Germany, especially those in which the percentage of mothers who breast-fed their babies was traditionally low (at least in the nineteenth century), the incidence and duration of breast-feeding increased. In the industrial conurbations, where more and more mothers were working, there was a marked improvement in dietary substitutes for infants after 1900. The increased availability of these was linked both to the rise in real incomes, which made prices more reasonable, and to the gradual dissemination of information explaining how such substitutes could be prepared, stored and served without risk to the infant's health.[55] On the other hand, it is less likely that the average standard of housing, at least in so far as hygiene was concerned, could have improved to such an extent that it affected the level of infant mortality, as Dickler assumes.[56] Thus, it was changes and improvements in the quality of the average diet that played a decisive and demonstrable role in bringing about a fall in infant mortality rates. However, the majority of the population remained unaffected until a relatively late stage because of the continued existence of a host of socio-cultural and economic obstacles — such as the numbers of working mothers (especially in rural districts), various traditional preferences for breast-feeding or artificial feeding, likewise traditional recipes and techniques used in preparing substitute babyfoods, average family sizes, and so on.

55. See Teuteberg and Bernhard, 'Wandel der Kindernahrung', pp. 183–97.
56. See Dickler, *Labour Market Pressure*, p. 214. For a recent and more detailed social history of housing conditions in the nineteenth century see H.-J. Teuteberg and C. Wischermann (eds), *Wohnalltag in Deutschland 1850–1914. Bilder-Daten-Dokumente* (Münster, 1985); H.-J. Teuteberg (ed.), *Homo Habitans. Zur Sozialgeschichte des ländlichen und städtischen Wohnens in der Neuzeit* (Münster, 1985). A statistical overview, which does, however, present some problems, is found in E. Gransche and F. Rothenbacher, 'Langfristige Entwicklungstendenzen der Wohnverhältnisse in Deutschland 1861–1910' (available as duplicated manuscript), SFB 3, Working Paper no. 158 (University of Mannheim, 1985); F. Rothenbacher, 'Soziale Ungleichheit des Wohnens in Deutschland im späten 19. und frühen 20. Jahrhundert' (available as duplicated manuscript), SFB 3, Working Paper no. 169 (University of Mannheim, 1985). For an exemplary analysis see C. Wischermann, *Wohnen in Hamburg vor dem Ersten Weltkrieg* (Münster, 1983). See also L. Niethammer (ed.), *Wohnen im Wandel* (Wuppertal, 1979); idem and F. Brüggemeier, 'Wie wohnten Arbeiter im Kaiserreich?', *Archiv für Sozialgeschichte*, 16 (1976), pp. 61–134.

6
Summary

Between 1870 and 1914, there was a marked expansion of the health sector, which was reflected in the rapid growth in the quality and quantity of facilities designed to combat ill-health, preserve the individual's ability to work for as long as possible, and, in the long term, provide more effective preventative care. In some fields — the construction of hospitals, for example — the level of provision of care grew dramatically after 1900, and there was initially actually a surplus of beds, relative to actual demand. The quantitative and qualitative improvements in services, including the introduction of statutory sickness (and disability) insurance, can be interpreted as a redistribution of the resources available for maintaining the health of the population as a whole. In view of certain restrictions on eligibility (especially for the benefits supported by the insurance funds) and the restricted access to certain institutions (particularly to the infrastructure that was, after all, concentrated in towns) the following groups seem to have been relatively deprived: women, infants, the elderly, unskilled and casual labourers, the unemployed, the disabled, beggars and tramps. Furthermore, there was also a perceptible trend towards changes that benefited the urban more than the rural population. The effects of the regional redistribution referred to above were reinforced by the process of internal migration that followed in the wake of industrialisation. Age structures in the new industrial conurbations meant that people tended to be healthier and fitter than in traditional and agricultural regions.

However, only a small part of the rather remarkable fall in the mortality rate — or, to put it differently, the improvement in the average life expectancy — can be attributed to advances made in medical science and the increased numbers of doctors, hospitals and hospital beds. Quite apart from the fact that there were broad regional variations in the way the facilities of the growing health sector were distributed, certain powerful social inhibitions also existed which, until the late nineteenth century, discouraged large sections of the working-class population from consulting a doctor or visiting a hospital when they fell ill, even when such facilities were available and within easy reach. However, the view that medical progress and the expanding health sector can be credited with no more than a fraction of the decline in the mortality rate is supported most convincingly by the fact that doctors simply lacked effective treatment for combating the 'great killers' of this period. In all probability, the relative number of deaths caused by certain widespread diseases such as tuberculosis, typhoid and whooping cough had already begun to fall by the beginning of the period I have been examining — that is, at a time when doctors still had no clear idea of their causes and the methods that might be used to combat them. As far as the other chronic and acute infectious diseases that began to decline from the early or mid-1880s are concerned, explanations must again be sought outside the field of curative medicine simply because real medical solutions, in the strict sense of the term, were not available (that is, apart from advice on diets and clothing, measures to improve public health and the health-related infrastructure).

If medical science did contribute in any meaningful way to the fall in the mortality rate, it was through advice and consultation rather than anything to do with treatment itself. The indisputable advances made in medical science from the 1860s onwards continued to have effects right into the early years of the twentieth century. Such progress placed developments in the field of public health and hygiene on a sure, scientific footing, with the result that authorities were encouraged to make more sizeable investments in the infrastructure and in the expansion of welfare facilities related to housing, employment and child- and mother-care. In addition, advances in medicine helped ensure that these developments were being organised and monitored in a systematic way, and guaranteed that facilities continued to function as efficiently as possible.

In this context, Pflanz has put forward the convincing argument that the decline of the infectious diseases

> must be understood in the context of the whole structure of social change: the intensification of health education, an environment favourable for public health, improvements in the quality of the average diet and workplace conditions, together with other manifestations of the improved standard of living all deserve mention in this respect.[57]

In actual fact, health education can only have occasioned a few very

---

57. M. Pflanz, *Sozialer Wandel und Krankheit. Ergebnisse und Probleme der medizinischen Soziologie* (Stuttgart, 1962), p. 172.

gradual changes in behaviour. These were probably connected with the campaigns organised in the first decade of the twentieth century to reduce the level of infant mortality, combat tuberculosis, reduce the housing shortage, fight alcoholism and improve the standards of domestic hygiene. At the same time, it is most likely that the health of a high percentage of those living in towns — with cities clearly leading the way — benefited from the rapid progress made in the field of urban sanitation. The process of infrastructural growth (the construction of central water supply and sewerage systems and the introduction of street-cleaning services, etc.) had demonstrably positive consequences in that it reduced the likelihood of infection in the cities and, in addition, encouraged the development of a more hygienic everyday environment. Of course, it should not be forgotten that the percentage of the total population that managed to derive any significant benefit from these developments was still rather small before 1900. Even in 1914, large sections of the populations of small towns and the majority of the rural population were largely excluded, though of course they did witness a decline in mortality and in the incidence of infectious diseases.

A further factor which must have had a positive impact on the 'nations's health' was the improvement in the standard of the average diet, which accompanied rises in real incomes from the 1870s onwards. The result was that physical resistance to germs and particularly to infectious diseases was likely to be greater. Other developments played a role too: real wages rose slowly but steadily; most people were able to take advantage of better-quality food supplies and to find relatively secure employment; the lower urban strata adapted more easily to the industrial and urban environment; and people lived their lives and expended their resources in a more rational manner. In those cases where the expansion of the health-related infrastructure exerted a direct influence, changes in the structure of unequally distributed social opportunities were reflected in the tendency for the relative positions of large social groups to converge. What is particularly striking is the considerable long-term benefit which accrued to the 'new middle class' in the wake of the effects which the health sector in the narrower — and the health-related infrastructure in the wider — sense had on life chances. But in addition to this, it is equally important to note that social differentiation within the working classes became much more marked, essentially between the skilled and unskilled; those who had assimilated urban life styles and those who had not; and, particularly with respect to the workers' movement, between organised and unorganised labour.[58] This, too, had consequences. It may therefore be said that market-determined class situations were modified both by processes of social stratification and by forces testifying to the power of overarching socio-cultural traditions. In turn, these modifications must have given rise to changes in relative market-determined positions in the network of social inequality, at least in the long term.

One significant influence on long-term changes in attitudes among large sections of the population, and on the deeper forces that gave rise to such changes, was the fact that the expansion of the health sector during this period was not solely a result of social and infrastructural policies implemented by the state: doctors and their professional organisations were also involved in instigating and organising the programme of expansion. Their efforts to achieve professional status, and, with the assistance of large sections of the educated strata, to medicalise the general public — and the lower classes in particular — must be regarded as instrumental in influencing the market capacities not only of doctors themselves, but also of the rest of the population. They proceeded to inject the modernisation process, which was to affect people's everyday lives, with forces that were to have a significant impact on public health standards and demographic developments, and in so doing played a part in creating, modifying and redistributing life chances. This will be discussed in greater detail in the next part of our study.

---

58. On these categories see W.H. Schröder, *Arbeitergeschichte und Arbeiterbewegung. Industriearbeit und Organisationsverhalten im 19. und frühen 20. Jahrhundert* (Frankfurt am Main and New York, 1978), pp. 41–50.

Part III
The Medicalisation of the Population, Professionalisation of Doctors, and Socio-Structural Change

7
A Theoretical Framework for an Analysis of Professionalisation

There is an almost perfect correlation between the major elements in the concept of professionalisation and the developmental stages in the history of the medical profession in industrial societies over the last century and a half. Both involve the occupational group gaining autonomy to decide on what is involved in the profession and how it is practised; regulating access to the profession and supervising the form and content of training; establishing the power to control the division of labour within the occupational field; organising the profession so it is able to bring pressure to bear as an interest group in the socio-political sphere; achieving the status of experts; and propagating a particular professional ethic. This is not entirely surprising when one considers that the professionalisation theory was extensively modelled on the example provided by developments in the medical profession.[1] While from a theoretical point of view, applying this concept in an investigation of physicians may appear to present some problems,[2] it does seem particularly appropriate if we are speaking of a socio-historical approach to the professionalisation of this group. This is also true of the only clear-cut criterion of professionalism, the group's socially legitimated autonomous control over what fell within the profession's ambit. A range of studies on developments

1. See E. Freidson, *Profession of Medicine. A Study of Sociology of Applied Knowledge* (New York, 1970), p. 4; on the concept of professionalisation, see ibid., p. 82.
2. See M. Sarfatti-Larson, *The Rise of Professionalism. A Sociological Analysis* (Berkley, 1977), pp. 37–8. In a similar vein, but for more detail on doctors in the nineteenth century, see G. Göckenjan, *Kurieren und Staat machen. Gesundheit und Medizin in der bürgerlichen Welt* (Frankfurt am Main, 1985); C. Huerkamp, 'Die preussisch-deutsche Ärzteschaft als Teil des Bildungsbürgertums: Wandel in Lage und Selbstverständnis vom ausgehenden 18. Jahrhundert bis zum Kaiserreich' in W. Conze and J. Kocka (eds), *Bildungsbürgertum im 19. Jahrhundert, vol. 1, Bildungsbürgertum und Professionalisierung in internationalen Vergleichen* (Stuttgart, 1985), pp. 358–87; idem, *Der Aufstieg der Ärzte*; M. Kater, 'Professionalization and Socialization of Physicians in Wilhelmine and Weimar Germany', *Journal of Contemporary History*, 20(4) (1985), pp. 677–701.

in the modern medical professions in the most varied societies shows that at the heart of the process by which they achieved professional autonomy lay a dual confrontation. On the one hand, they successfully confronted the state which attempted to intervene excessively in affairs, and, on the other, they limited the competitive power of other social groups traditionally concerned with health and illness.

An interesting way of developing this approach further is to assess an occupational group's chances of professionalisation by establishing to what extent it is successful in creating a market outlet for its services and of gaining monopoly control over them as a profession.[3] To achieve this, the services (i.e. the products) of the group seeking professionalisation must be standardised in such a way that potential competitors can be excluded from the market. In the case of doctors, a number of factors, which were combined in varying ways from country to country, assisted in this process. For example, hospitals were developing (which in particular went to link up patient care, medical research and training); doctors as a group were in close contact with the development of medical science and progress in medical technology; medical training was being centralised and monopolised in universities; and the belief that doctors contributed to the general welfare was being cultivated. To these factors must be added a decisive condition for ensuring success, the necessity of evoking in the public mind an awareness of the exclusive abilities of doctors to cure efficiently just what needed curing, i.e. the belief in the superiority of doctors in diagnosing and treating diseases. A profession can only ensure a genuine monopoly of its services and consequently enjoy an autonomy sanctioned by society after such a belief has taken root. As a prerequisite of success, this involves consolidating and, in the long term, expanding a clearly defined market for medical services which the profession can control by excluding competitors or at least subjecting them to regulation.

By taking as an example the professionalisation of doctors in late nineteenth and early twentieth century Germany, some indication will be given below of what form this process actually took in its particular historical setting. At the same time, we shall attempt to establish the significance of medical professionalisation for long-term changes in social structure. In doing so, areas which on the whole are regularly broached by sociological investigations of professionalisation (for example displacing 'competition', the 'ex-

---

3. See Sarfatti-Larson, *The Rise*, pp. 20–5, 35–7.

propriation of health') will only be touched upon, while the main emphasis will thus be on aspects which have been somewhat neglected hitherto and which can be seen collectively as the contribution doctors made to the medicalisation of German society.

8
Medical Reforms and the Suppression of Lay Healers in the Mid-Nineteenth Century

The situation of doctors in mid-nineteenth-century German society was recently described as follows:

> The comparatively backward state of medical research meant that relatively little scientific knowledge was expected of the individual doctor who was mainly a practical man. In most cases individual doctors were able to keep a more or less firm grasp on the most important areas of their subject . . . The doctor had a fixed clientele which hardly ever fluctuated. A doctor's behaviour was conceived in terms of 'consciously authoritarian, patriarchal care' . . . Doctors in the nineteenth century were thus characterised by professional autonomy and autarchy, an income commensurate with others in their status-group and a highly prestigious position.[4]

By constrast, Claudia Huerkamp, whose results will be referred to below, painted the following picture of doctors in the first half of the nineteenth century:

> Doctors did not form a unitary occupational group but fell into a number of extremely heterogenous groups which in turn can be divided roughly into two parts. The great majority were not academics but had at best undergone some kind of practical training. They were surgeons, barbers and barber-surgeons of varying levels of skill. The smaller group, the 'educated doctors', had indeed attended university medical faculties, but medical knowledge at the time was mainly symptom-orientated and speculative, with the success of any treatment highly uncertain and at times more a matter of luck than judgement. Thus it cannot be concluded that doctors had expert knowledge based on specialist training which might have guaranteed that they were techni-

---

4. F. Naschold, *Kassenärzte und Krankenversicherungsreform. Zu einer Theorie der Statuspolitik* (Freiburg, 1967) pp. 90–3.

cally superior to competitors offering medical services. Where individual doctors enjoyed high social prestige it was not due to their medical expertise but rather to their social background, their connections and their general education which elevated them to the ranks of the 'educated classes'.[5]

This is still to leave out of account the large number of lay healers whose clientele came from the lower strata, and particularly from the rural areas where there was a shortage of any kind of qualified doctors. These were, for example, fortune-tellers, exorcists, charmers who promised to drive the devil from the soul, alchemists, priests, lay brothers and sisters, midwives, old wise women, nuns and monks, 'piss prophets' and others. Given the unstructured coexistence of the most varied groups offering health services, it was impossible for one small subgroup, doctors who had undergone academic education, to establish professional autonomy in the absence of recognised and identifiable expert knowledge.

In the first half of the nineteenth century, however, almost all large German states witnessed attempts to unify doctors into one status group. While these efforts were occasionally supported by certain groups of doctors pursuing particular interests (for example, educated doctors distancing themselves more clearly from those below, or less qualified surgeons raising their social status), the driving force was provided by state-led initiatives and constant interest shown by the state in having a medical infrastructure that would be qualitatively better and at the same time easier to control (in the sense of traditional medical policing). Here we must bear in mind the status or virtual status of doctors as state officials until trade restrictions (including those for pathology) were lifted by the 1869 Trade Act of the North German Confederation, and the 1871 Trade Act of the German Empire. For example, after the Decree on Medicine (*Medizinalordnung*) of 1806 in the Grand Duchy of Baden, all those occupied in medicine (doctors, senior surgeons, junior surgeons, midwives, apothecaries) held the 'position of public health official' (*die Stellung von öffentlichen Gesundheitsbeamten*).[6] Private doctors also had this quasi-official status in Prussia until 1869.[7] Given this structure of pre-modern health care

---

5. Huerkamp, 'Ärzte', pp. 350–1. See also P.U. Unschuld, 'Professionalisierung und ihre Folgen' in H. Schipperges et al. (eds), *Krankheit, Heilkunst, Heilung* (Freiburg and Munich, 1978), p. 530.
6. *Bericht des Großherzoglichen Obermedizinalraths an Großherzogliches Ministerium des Innern über den Zustand des Medizinalwesens im Großherzogthum Baden im Jahre 1869* (Karlsruhe, 1871), p. 39.
7. See Huerkamp, 'Ärzte', pp. 361ff.

and the configuration of interests we have mentioned, medical practitioners could not have been unified into one group through a process by which educated doctors imposed a monopoly, as professionalisation theory would suppose. Rather, the latter had first of all to integrate (or be integrated) with some of the lower categories of doctors, a process which generally went hand in hand with a reform of university training courses by which standards of qualifications were set at a uniformly higher level. The larger number of academics which resulted were now able to dominate other practitioners, who were bound to remain unequivocally subordinate as long as the state controlled training courses or issued professional licences. For example, in Prussia from 1852 onwards medical assistants (*Heildiener*) and midwives had to pass state examinations and hold a state licence to practise, as did hospital nurses later on.

From the beginning of the nineteenth century until the Trade Acts of 1869 and 1871, which lifted some restrictions on healing practices, two main developments occurred in the medical occupations in the larger German states. Firstly, the number of different occupations decreased, that is health care became homogenous; and secondly, three subgroups of practitioners emerged each with a different status. On the one hand, there were two groups of trained practitioners who were licensed by the state. Among these, graduate doctors, who by now included qualified surgeons, enjoyed a distinctly superior status. On the other hand, there were the lay healers (increasingly referred to collectively as 'quacks'), to some extent discriminated against and threatened by criminal law and the police. It must be emphasised however that 'the state bureaucracy initiated the transformation of the pattern of premodern medicine, the main feature of which was the existence of various subgroups differentiated by the social background, education and status of their members, and by their contact with particular types of clientele.'[8] Part of the reason why the state played such a major role in the process, in contrast to what happened in the USA and Britain for example, lay in the fact that 'in Germany even before the traditional roles of doctors were modernised, the state controlled and financed the training institutions and appointed the examining boards.'[9]

From an initial examination it may be surmised that all this must have had considerable consequences for structures of social in-

8. Ibid., p. 360.
9. Ibid., p. 361.

equality. Above all, these developments reveal tendencies which were not to have their full impact until the following decades, which is to say the period I am investigating. The most striking changes occurred in the structure of health care and health services. The integration of internal medicine, surgery and obstetrics had meant that graduate doctors were now subject to the same processes of socialisation and enjoyed the same status. Their prestige rose to such a degree that the establishment of uniformity in this area can be interpreted as a stage in collective upward social mobility. The group also presumably became more exclusive in terms of social origins as a result of more exacting entry qualifications (secondary school examination in the humanities) and the need to have completed university studies. Consequently other healers who subsequently came to be regarded as inferior lost out to doctors and were subjected to their dominance. This was a remarkable process to the extent that it was by no means underpinned either by generally accepted advances in medical science or even by socially recognised improvements in the physician's ability to diagnose and treat illnesses between the 1850s and the 1870s.

It is rather the case that medical treatment around the middle of the nineteenth century was characterised by a 'crisis of confidence which followed the therapeutic chaos of those years'.[10] The ironic tones of a contemporary doctor are indicative of this:

> In the olden days doctors were glad if they only had one cure for every illness, and they hadn't got any at all for many. We're much better off! Not only do we have vast numbers of medicines for every single illness, but every single medicine cures vast numbers of illnesses. However, the real triumph of science is that now we have the most powerful medicines against the most incurable illnesses, . . . and as far as I can recall, all of them have been absolutely infallible.'[11]

The great mass of the population must have thus put more trust in the healing powers of those who came from a similar social background and who had traditionally proved their worth. It can be assumed that the social elites (aristocracy and upper-middle classes) also mistrusted the state of medical science and practice since it in no way guaranteed that graduate doctors were actually better at curing illnesses. Even if doctors were to some extent privileged by the social elites and granted the first stages of professional auton-

---

10. C.v. Ferber, *Soziologie für Mediziner. Eine Einführung* (Berlin, 1975), p. 14.
11. Fechner, cited by E.H. Ackerknecht, *Therapie von den Primitiven bis zum 20. Jahrhundert* (Stuttgart, 1970), p. 122.

omy (particularly in contrast to the inferior groups in health care), the main explanation for their rise to dominance must primarily be sought in the interests of state bureaucracy and the power it exercised through its policing function.

'The high status of doctors before systems of social security were introduced resulted thus not from privileges derived from their occupational role, but to a large degree from the power structure of the society of the day which was dysfunctional for society's health needs on the whole.'[12] Against this background it can be seen that insofar as doctors as part of the educated bourgeoisie were now being granted higher social status as symbolic compensation for the past, probably as a reaction to the social reformism and revolutionary movements in the bourgeoisie of the 1840s, the process by which doctors were unified into a status group and began to enjoy relative privilege was power-related. However, a more important reason must have been that medical reforms made it much easier to monitor and control the infrastructure by way of medical policing (for example, fighting plagues, use of quarantine, care for the poor). The pre-democratic (monarchist) German states did not need experts in medical science, nor those with obviously superior healing powers, to fulfil this purpose and ensure that the symbolic power of the relevant social institutions was maintained. It was much more the case that as far as the state was concerned the occupational group involved had to be able to exercise the authority invested in it by the sovereign institutions in a socially acceptable manner, and remain numerically small enough to be manageable. The state also needed to be directly involved in training and recruitment in order to monitor its activities. These factors, and not the (lack of) expert knowledge which many sociologists regard as the occupation's dominant feature, characterised the professional role of doctors in the middle of the century and explain the state's interest in granting them privileges.

Another significant element of the changes in structures of social inequality we have been describing concerns the large groups of people involved in health care who, together with the traditional forms and practices of medicine they represented, lost status and tended to be regarded as criminals. A categorical concomitant of the socio-structural changes generated by capitalist industrialisation and urbanisation is a progressive decline among large social groups in their first-hand knowledge and experience of nature and the human body. In addition, the long-term evolution of modern

12. Naschold, 'Kassenärzte', p. 94.

science induces natural scientists to rationalise and monopolise the areas of knowledge in which they are experienced. This tendency was appreciably reinforced by state medical reforms in mid-nineteenth-century Germany, for these entailed a rise in status for graduate doctors, and a loss of status for those practising other forms of health care, some of which even became illegal.[13] These reforms put doctors in a position from which they would be able to monopolise the superior medical knowledge they were later to gain. The result was that large sections of the lower strata tended to become less and less acquainted with traditional medical lore and the related forms of self-help. Here are the first signs of what, in the light of subsequent developments, was termed the 'expropriation of health'. It is of particular importance that until 1869–71 those practising various forms of lay healing ('quackery') were threatened with punishment. The point is that, even after the general ban on 'quacks' was lifted, many forms of diagnosis and treatment which were entirely worthy of consideration yet discredited by the 'medical school' could not shake off their reputation of being illegal and second-class. In view of the extremely low number of doctors per head of population, especially in rural areas — a situation which remained unchanged throughout the nineteenth century despite certain improvements — and considering the cultural and financial barriers which excluded large parts of the population from the possibility of consulting a doctor, even if one could be found in the area, one must conclude that the medical reforms around the middle of the nineteenth century led to a deterioration in health care and consultation among the lower urban strata and in the rural population as a whole. Here, too, the long-term consequences of the course embarked upon are more important than its short-term effects, which in all probability were barely felt by the majority of people at the time.

13. See, for example, Ottmüller, 'Speikinder'; idem, 'Mutterpflichten'; Freidson, 'Profession', p. 371; Unschuld, 'Professionalisierung', pp. 530–1; I. Illich, *Medical Nemesis. The Expropriation of Health* (London, 1975).

9
Integration of Competing Interests, Resistance to Social Regulation, and Professionalisation

In the 1870s circumstances for German doctors changed in a way which even in retrospect is quite striking.

> At the instigation of Deputies of the North German Reichstag, who were doctors and who referred to a petition presented by the Berlin Medical Society, medicine . . . was declared a trade which anyone could practise. . . . Only the title 'Doctor' remained protected: individuals who did not hold a state licence to practise were barred from using this or a similar title. This new version of §29 of the Trade Act simultaneously annulled §199 and §200 of the Prussian Criminal Code. In addition the official oath became obsolete as did the right of the medical authorities to withdraw a doctor's licence to practise.[14]

The new conditions amounted to a kind of exchange in that both the legal obligation of doctors to treat urgent cases (*Kurierzwang*) (§200) and the ban on 'quacks' were repealed. In other words, doctors relinquished some of their legal privileges, particularly since the new system formally removed unregistered medical practices from the realm of illegality. The fact that it was doctors who had insisted that the ban on 'quacks' was abolished and had thus sacrificed their own privileges contradicts all the normal assumptions of the professionalisation theory. On this point, Claudia Huerkamp remarks that, for one thing, the Berlin doctors who took the initiative were convinced that the ban was actually ineffective. For another, they were among the elite doctors (and included a large number of university professors) and thus had a clientele far out of the reach of any lay practitioners.

In all probability such great confidence on the part of the Berlin Medical Society and their lack of fear of competition from lay healers reflected a new trend. In contrast to what had traditionally

14. Huerkamp, 'Ärzte', p. 364.

been the case, the confidence cannot have been derived from the social prestige of the clientele or from establishment-approved authority, but from the direct effects of two developments which were not fully recognised by doctors and by the general public until the following decades: considerable progress in medical science; and the tangible successes (although these were partly exaggerated by propaganda) of campaigns for improved sanitation and public health in which doctors played a major part. The two developments strengthened the authority of doctors in the eyes of both the state and society and were conducive in the long term to their achieving the status of experts.

However the united step forward taken by the doctors of Berlin surprised the vast majority of their colleagues and was by no means uncontroversial. Clearly those in the elite advocating progress in medical science and in social and political affairs, most of whom were politically liberal in the 1860s and 1870s, were opposed by a majority who by contrast were further removed from science and politics and who subscribed rather to conservative social doctrines. This conflict of interest does not seem to have had any identifiable political significance during the period under investigation. Other areas of contention were more important and led to confrontation among doctors. The crucial innovation brought about by the Trade Act must have been not so much the abolition of the legal obligations and the ban on 'quacks', which were so frequently discussed in later years, but the connected effect of a clear end to state supervision over the medical profession. (The legal obligations of §200, it must be said, did reappear in a slightly modified form later on when doctors created their own Ethical Committees — (*Ehrenräte*.) Only in the course of the 1880s and 1890s, when further factors, to be discussed below, came into play, did doctors realise the ambivalent consequences of releasing medical practice from regulation from above, and of the resultant establishment of free market conditions in the health sector. These effects began to be felt when it transpired that doctors were competing against each other and possibly also against 'quacks', which may have threatened the maintenance of income levels, especially for some members of the status group. It was not until changes in the labour market gradually led to difficulties in maintaining incomes that the underlying causes of these developments occupied the attention of doctors more. If it is, in fact, a significant factor, it seems possible that income levels began to be threatened in this way in the late 1880s. From that time onwards, the fight against 'quacks', in other words the fight to establish a standard product and hence a legitimate, unified group offering that product, was at its fiercest.

Before examining the particular developments in the 1880s and 1890s, we should look at an aspect of the liberalisation of the medical profession, which was important for professionalisation, even though in retrospect doctors tend not to emphasise it. What happened was that alongside

> a cut-back in state supervision of doctors ... the role of medical associations became more important. After an initial boom in the number of these groups, which went through a period of temporary politicisation in the 1840s ... a further spate of such organisations appeared in the second half of the 1860s. Then in 1873 the Federation of Medical Associations (*Ärztevereinsbund*) was formed as an umbrella organisation, and the annual medical conferences held from then on became important channels for propagating the group interests of doctors. In addition to pressing for continuous training, representing their members' interests and also having a say on medical affairs in public and in dealings with the health authorities, medical associations began more and more to set out rules for doctors in 'Codes of Professional Conduct' and to ensure these were observed through 'Ethical Committees' or similar committees. This professional structure and the transformation of medical associations from loose-knit organisations fulfilling primarily scientific and social functions into efficient organs of interest representation are equally as important for the professionalisation of doctors as the unification of the occupational group which was achieved by standardising training and reducing bureaucratic state intervention.[15]

Three fundamental changes in the labour market for doctors in the late nineteenth century accelerated this process of professionalisation: the introduction of statutory sickness insurance in 1883, the rapid rise in the number of doctors from the end of the 1880s onwards (i.e. the growth in the number of medical students), and increasingly tangible progress in medical science and technology.

The socio-structural significance of the developments which occurred at the beginning of our period should be seen in the context of emerging clashes of interest and status among doctors. Lines of conflict were drawn between doctors whose patients were covered by sickness insurance and those whose patients were not insured, and between general practitioners and consultants. The rift between the latter was less marked, but nevertheless important in the long run. Conflicts of interests also came to a head between hospital doctors and private practitioners, on the one hand, and

15. Ibid., pp. 366–7.

between doctors in the town and the country on the other. However, it turned out that right up to the First World War doctors managed increasingly to ensure that all these conflicts, which did occasionally lead to serious disputes, and the considerable disparities in working conditions, income levels, social status and overall life chances which underlay them, remained matters dealt with entirely within the confines of the profession. The conflicts did not slow down the process of the unification of doctors as a status group, either formally or in terms of their ability to represent their interests in society. In fact the profession appeared to be a relatively cohesive unit acting on behalf of all doctors. All this must have been an effect of legislation on social security which had unintended, though far-reaching, consequences.

The literature frequently emphasises that after the introduction of the Sickness Insurance Act the market for the services offered by doctors grew noticeably. (We shall return to this below.) It was helped by the long-term increase in real wages for the lower social strata, on the one hand, and by changes in life style occasioned by urbanisation on the other. Less attention has been paid to how from the beginning of the 1890s onwards doctors for the first time 'became aware of themselves' as a profession in the real sense as a result of confrontation with sickness insurance funds which were becoming ever more important. The 'forced' expansion of the market was perceived in terms of much tougher competition, greater polarisation of — and ultimately a threat to — status. The cohesion of the professional group grew commensurately and was reflected in the way in which the medical associations organised and discussed their affairs: the issue of scientific and technical modernisation was included in a reform of the health sector and of university medical studies and presented to the public in the form of demands for more advanced medical care. A professional ethos (a status-group ideology) which served a strategic purpose as the doctor's trademark was evolved and put into practice with favourable results for the doctors' public image. There were two sides to this acceleration of professionalisation. It fused modernisation and demands for progress with demands which opposed the free market economy, were more traditional and designed to boost doctors' status. It can be viewed as an example of how status-group politics attempt to counteract the dynamics of class formation. These decisive stages in the professionalisation of German doctors took the form of initially spontaneous and practical efforts to fight off the threat, as doctors perceived it, of the challenge posed by the sickness insurance funds and the labour movement controlling them.[16] One sign of the contradictory face of professionalisation is the fact that the interests of the status group in re-establishing former privileges and resisting pressures for social regulation of the health sector were consciously pursued using trade union methods such as strikes, boycotts, and tightening up internal ideology and control.

16. See A. Labisch, 'Ärzte und Arbeiterbewegung', *Medizinsoziologische Mitteilungen*, 3(4) (1977), p. 13.

10
Resistance to Monopolisation of the Medical Market by Doctors

Despite many other victories won by doctors in the early part of the twentieth century in the struggle to fight off the threat — as they saw it — that health services and their profession would be subject to social regulation, they did not manage to restore the legally sanctioned monopoly they had enjoyed before the introduction of liberalisation. It is clear that before the First World War doctors were unable to convince either the public or the ruling elites of the need for such privilege (i.e. a ban on 'quacks'). It was not the presumed (though at no point proven) drop in income as a result of competition from lay healers which was the bitter pill for doctors to swallow; even less was it the damage they complained had been done to the honour of the profession by the shady and at times even blatantly criminal practices of some 'quacks'. It was much more the fact that doctors' demands for a monopoly over medical treatment were not recognised either in the first round of sickness insurance legislation in 1883 nor in subsequent amendments. Indeed, during the late nineteenth and early twentieth centuries sickness insurance funds occasionally even remunerated 'quacks'. While there has never been any detailed evidence on the extent of this practice, medical associations vehemently protested against it, citing various examples to support their case. It became possible after the Trade Act had lifted restrictions on medical occupations, and because formulations in the sickness insurance legislation were vague: §6 stated that from the contraction of illness the patient should among other things be guaranteed free medical treatment.

Following a parliamentary question from the medical associations in the Reichstag in 1887, Minister of State von Boetticher took a most informative line on contemporary interpretations of the controversial term 'medical treatment'. He explained that the wording of the legislation did not explicitly 'state that only doctors are permitted to practise the art of medicine. "Medical treatment" means treatment of illness in general. If only doctors were to be allowed to treat those covered by sickness insurance, then the wording of the law would have to be changed'.[17] But as von Boetticher went on to spell out, an amendment to the law was entirely out of the question for the reason that many members of the public who required medical treatment still preferred to turn to healers who were not doctors but whom they none the less trusted. This situation did not change in its legal aspects until after the First World War. It does seem possible, however, that doctors were gradually able to get sickness insurance funds to agree at least in practice that medical treatment should only be administered by licensed doctors.

This makes the doctor's strategy of discrediting lay healers by using every available method of propaganda all the more understandable. A typical statement on this problem is to be found in the 1901 Medical Report for the Prussian State: 'Given the conceited arrogance and usually unscrupulous and unconscientious practices of a large number of these most inferior and dubious characters indulging in quackery, it is no wonder that the damage they inflict on life and health is considerable.'[18] No solid evidence was offered to support such acerbic generalisations. It was usually enough to mention a few lay healers who had previous convictions for theft and immoral conduct.

It is not only the relatively large number of 'quacks', which was discussed in Chapter 3 above, which suggests that even by the beginning of the twentieth century the authority of professional medicine was still barely respected by the wider population, especially in rural regions. In addition, whole areas of medicine such as natural healing were favoured over other forms. These methods, which were developed and practised outside 'official medicine' presumably had to be fought against so strongly because during the period under investigation they more and more rapidly became established among the wider population as a kind of reaction to signs of industrialisation in medicine and pharmacology. Advocates of these methods, who as such were in competition with

---

17. C. von Littrow, 'Die Stellung des Deutschen Ärztetages zur Kurpfuscherfrage in Deutschland von 1869 bis 1908', *Wissenschaftliche Zeitschrift der Humboldt-Universität zu Berlin*, Mathematisch-Naturwissenschaftliche Reihe, *19*(4) (1970), p. 439. For a more detailed account see idem, 'Der Deutsche Ärztetag und die Kurpfuscherfrage. (Ein Beitrag zur Geschichte der Kurpfuscherei in Deutschland von 1869 bis 1908)' (unpubl. diss., Humboldt-Universität, Berlin, 1969), pp. 74–86.
18. *Das Gesundheitswesen des Preußischen Staates im Jahre 1901*, p. 495. On the reactions of the discriminated parties, see Zentralverband für Parität der Heilmethoden (eds), *Schriften über Wesen und Bedeutung der Kurierfreiheit*, first series, nos 1–6 (Berlin, 1911).

professional doctors, included, it would appear, 'religious healers, artisans, nurses (*Heildiener*), barber-surgeons, herbalists, shepherds, and failed students'. A particularly vigorous propaganda campaign was launched against school teachers who tried to 'discredit scientific medicine' in public lectures or by organising 'associations for the cultivation of natural healing' (*Vereine zur Pflege der Naturheilverfahren*). This evidence leads me to proffer the hypothesis that attempts to impose a monopoly by doctors on the medical market, which would fit in with professionalisation theory, were in fact unsuccessful before the First World War (with the exception of some peripheral areas such as inoculation, forensic medicine, certain advisory functions in the public sector). I would contend that the main reason for this was that science-based medicine did begin to command greater respect during the period we are examining, but on the whole did not spread to sufficiently large sections of the population, and certainly did not proceed unchallenged.

Medical science and technology had been progressing in leaps and bounds since the late 1860s, as had pharmacology. Discoveries and developments allowed licensed doctors to diagnose and treat illnesses on a new, improved basis akin to the normal procedure of natural science of testing and verifying hypotheses. As a result, medical science was now in a better position to demonstrate to the public that its achievements were based upon findings which could be checked by other members of the scientific community, which satisfied the methodological standards of strict science and which were thus open to reasoned reflection and inquiry. But this did not automatically mean that educated doctors were able to secure a generally better position in the market for selling their services. The difficulty they faced was that up until the last years of the nineteenth century legitimation of an activity by natural science did not in any way mean that every social group and subculture ascribed to it an equal or even higher value (in contrast to traditional forms of legitimation). This was compounded by the fact that, by the end of the nineteenth century, only very few areas of therapy had yielded verifiable and universally recognised results. New findings (for example in microbiology and bacteriology) and new techniques (such as the introduction of X-rays and serodiagnosis) may have placed diagnosis on a firmer basis, but only rarely did it lead directly to improvements in therapy. As far as this did occur, it was primarily in the field of hospital treatment (obstetrics, and the discovery and application of anaesthetics, antiseptics and aseptics in surgery), the reputation of which thus grew rapidly in the later decades of the nineteenth century. As far as our period is concerned, however, it was only the rare exception among the mass of established doctors who offered a medical service superior to that of lay healers.

The formation and consolidation of the medical profession must be seen as being closely connected with the evolving structure of a clearly defined market for doctors' services, and with the way in which society's trust in and recognition of doctors led this market to expand to the detriment of traditional forms of healing. This two-sided process should be understood as part of the secular socio-structural changes which an industrialising society undergoes. Industrialisation and urbanisation were bound up with radical changes in social structure which not only created entirely new living conditions for continually expanding sections of the population, brought about a fundamental change in value systems, endowed the lower social strata with greater purchasing power, and induced processes of class formation which reshaped traditional patterns of social stratification. The changes objectively favoured the demand for services offered by licensed doctors, whose share of the market should have grown at the expense of other suppliers of health services. But this growth had still not taken place in the early 1880s. In fact, the number of doctors grew at an even slower rate than the population, in other words slower than the potential demand. Until this point doctors failed to break into areas of the market fixed by subcultural boundaries. For this to happen, perceptions of health and illness and thus the norms governing consumption of the product offered by doctors had to be generalised. In other words, certain ideas and norms had to be accepted by society as a whole such that a particular product (doctors' services) would be in demand irrespective of subcultural mentalities. A considerably larger market for medical services, unfettered by traditional attitudes to health and illness and free of the influence of traditional healing practices, had to be established, which would seem both attractive and legitimate to the great majority of the population.

As a single occupational group, doctors would never have been able to generate social changes as comprehensive as the replacement of the orientations and life style of specific groups by values and norms shared by all sectors of society. But doctors did objectively — i.e. unconsciously — take the requirements of this process into consideration, by insisting from the 1870s onwards that professional training and practice conformed more and more to standards which could be scientifically tested and legitimated. From this angle, new light is thrown on doctors' attempts to overcome what looked like a saturation of the profession in the 1880s and 1890s by, among other things, extending the length of training and raising the standards required for qualification. Although even in the long term these attempts did not manage to prevent the number of medical students rising in absolute and relative terms — in this sense they represented a fairly unsuccessful labour market strategy — they did accelerate the way in which scientific research and technical innovation were beginning to give doctors authority and a superior position in the medical market. Standardisation, so to speak, of suppliers (i.e. doctors), through scientific and professional methods of supervising training, examinations and, ultimately, access to the occupation meant that scientific criteria were also being used to make the market for medical services uniform and legitimate. In the long term this was to be an important condition for other suppliers to lose effective status and be pushed out of the market which doctors increasingly came to dominate.

The fight against 'quackery' mentioned above which, due to the lack of support from the state, was conducted in collaboration with the medical associations, their publications and special campaigns, is evidence that, right up until the end of our period, the direct attacks launched by doctors on the underlying norms of the areas of the medical market they had yet to penetrate were ineffective. Many doctors were aware that the numerous sectors of the medical market were relatively distinct from each other. There was only negligible direct competition between lay healers and doctors, for example, which affected income levels.[19] Other groups of doctors,

19. The reasons given by the Berlin Medical Gesellschaft (*Berliner Medizinische Gesellschaft*) for their demand to have the ban on 'quacks' lifted can be interpreted in this way; see Huerkamp, 'Ärzte', pp. 363ff. Two opposing statements of the day illustrate clearly the difference of opinion on the significance of 'quackery' for the status and income of doctors. Having complained of the growth in the number of 'quacks' and the damage they had caused to public health, Dr Aschenborn, speaking for Prussian medical officials, came to the conclusion that 'doctors have suffered professionally from this too. Take reputations, for one thing. For the general public, undiscerning as it usually tends to be, the difference between doctor and quack lost the clarity the law once so unequivocally gave to it, and became so indistinct that people began to regard doctors and quacks as equals, without judging the activities of one to be superior to those of the other. It is just the same for incomes. The vast sums of money accruing to quacks each year mean losses for doctors, who are forced to take a significant cut in their incomes' (Aschenborn, 'Ärzte', p. 373). Contrast this with Plaut: 'In addition there is the question of whether in fact quacks actually do fully compete with doctors. The answer must be no . . . For one thing, in the regions with few doctors, those which are not able to support a doctor, an old, experienced shepherd will be able to make his living by working as a quack now and again, and for another the treatment administered by 'unlicensed individuals' is often so eccentric that one is convinced doctors could only benefit from as many of these people as possible' (T. Plaut, *Der Gewerkschaftskampf der deutschen Ärzte* (Karlsruhe, 1913), p. 75, (no. 14 of new series of *Volkswirtschaftliche Abhandlungen der badischen Hochschulen*)).

not least the Prussian Medical Administration, presumably felt that the danger lay much more at the level of norms and values. The dislocated nature of the market for medical services was after all an indication that specific norms and perceptions of health and illness and hence greatly differing forms of treatment were to be found in various subcultures. This threatened the market share held by doctors to the extent that it called into question their underlying values, based as they were on universalist assumptions, and cast aspersions particularly on the validity of science in legitimating doctors' services.[20] From this point of view, the 'fight against quackery', which was fairly ineffective as a labour market strategy in purely quantitative terms, takes on an ideological significance very much worth discussing, even though its efficacy is difficult to assess.

It was doubtless the complex process of social change as a whole which effectively generated increasing needs throughout society for the services provided by doctors and which led to the adoption of norms which in turn legitimated these needs. Notwithstanding this, it should not be forgotten that doctors undertook a whole series of activities which reinforced and even distinctly shaped social change in such a way as to promote their profession. The action taken by doctors on infrastructure policy and social security which, as it rapidly expanded, gradually took on the characteristics of a system, is most pertinent here. But even more important perhaps was the social position doctors acquired after the introduction of statutory sickness insurance, since this legislation provided a legally binding definition of what role health and illness should play in the labour market. If we wish to find a term to describe these developments, which led to a relatively rapid expansion of the share of the medical market dominated by licensed doctors from the 1880s onwards, then we might talk of medicalisation.[21] This refers to all developments which favoured positive attitudes to health, illness and science-based medicine in conjunction with the

20. See Sarfatti-Larson, *The Rise*, pp. 20–1, 25, 35. For more details see Huerkamp and Spree, 'Arbeitsmarktstrategien', section 3.
21. On the historical context which led Foucault to propagate the concept of medicalisation as the change in mentality in Europe from the late eighteenth century onwards that resulted from the steps taken by health authorities and from policy initiatives on health and population, see the introduction to A.E. Imhof (ed.), *Biologie des Menschen in der Geschichte* (Stuttgart-Bad Cannstatt, 1978), pp. 62–75. The multifarious concept simultaneously comprises the traditional component of intervention in the health or ill-health of the individual by established authority, or by a body which is legitimated by state and society (the modern term being 'expropriation of health'), and the other, ambivalent, component of individual rationalisation of reproductive behaviour in line with the modernisation of society.

spread of rationalist value-systems and forms of behaviour, particularly in private life, the displacement of traditional behavioural orientations fixed in subcultures, and the adoption by society in general of bourgeois norms. Considering that the majority of social groups very much kept their distance from doctors and the medical institutions of the infrastructure until the late nineteenth century, it would seem important to look more closely at the mechanisms of medicalisation at work in these sections of the population.

11
'Enforced Socialisation' of the Lower Classes and Medicalisation

Opposition to the efforts made by the practitioners of scientifically based medicine to monopolise medical treatment came mainly from two groups: the rural population and the working class. The former hardly ever came into contact with the actual or presumed successes of modern medicine. The distance to the nearest doctor, low incomes and the absence of insurance to a large degree led people to administer their own medical treatment. They drew on their own experience (including that gained by dealing with animals) and traditional books, used customary domestic drugs and forms of care, and turned for assistance to the traditional healers from their own social milieu. Little of this changed before the First World War.[22] It was the cultural distance from academic and professional medicine, reliance on traditional forms of treatment and above all the lack of financial resources which placed a block between the working class and doctors. In the face of widespread poverty, lack of future prospects, and social dislocation, it is likely that the working class and the lower urban strata for a long time adopted a generally fatalistic attitude towards illness and affliction. Under these circumstances the emerging institutions of social security, increasingly structured as systems, and above all the Sickness Insurance Act, presumably acted like a process of 'prescribed social learning', as von Ferber terms it, the effect of which might be called 'enforced socialisation'.[23] Even if it was for motives which

22. See, for example, Shorter, *Bedside Manners*, pp. 55–74; von Ferber, *Soziologie*, p. 40; Huerkamp, *Der Aufstieg der Ärzte*, chapter 2.
23. See von Ferber, *Soziologie*, pp. 44–8; for the theoretical framework see ibid., pp. 55–63. Ute Frevert assumes similar effects were produced by the early factory sickness insurance funds; see U. Frevert, 'Arbeiterkrankheit und Arbeiterkrankenkassen im Industrialisierungsprozess Preussens (1840–1870)' in W. Conze and E. Engelhardt, *Arbeiterexistenz*, esp. pp. 303–8; idem, 'Professional Medicine and the Working Classes in Imperial Germany', *Journal of Contemporary History*, 20(4) (1985), pp. 637–58; idem, '"Fürsorgliche Belagerung": Hygienebewegung und Arbeiterfrauen im 19. und frühen 20. Jahrhundert', *Geschichte und Gesellschaft*, 11(4) (1985), pp. 420–46; idem, *Krankheit als politisches Problem 1770–1880. Soziale Unterschichten in Preussen zwischen medizinischer Polizei und staatlicher Sozialversicherung*

rarely coincided with the thinking behind official social policy, 'prescribed social learning' was supported by the organised labour movement, particularly in so far as it concerned health care and the use of infrastructural services.

In this final section, the way in which the medicalisation of the lower strata manifested itself as 'enforced socialisation' will be examined in slightly more detail because it produced very important long-term changes in the pattern of structural social inequality, although these were perhaps not immediately visible to society at the time. There is also a direct link with the professionalisation of doctors, since we can regard this partly as a process by which an occupational group followed a strategy of actively influencing class formation to its own advantage.

Towards the end of the nineteenth and particularly in the early twentieth centuries, the totality of social institutions and measures we have mentioned gradually lost the character of a collection of isolated, uncoordinated initiatives, so that it becomes more apt to speak of the establishment of a system. Beyond fulfilling its immediate purpose, the emerging system of social controls and security had — and this is the crucial question — the function of setting in motion what we have called 'prescribed social learning', especially for the lower classes. Private, charitable bourgeois organisations were originally responsible for many of the measures which are of relevance here. In the late nineteenth century it was typical for these to overlap with or be augmented by state activities, acquire official status or even be taken over by the state. This development is merely a reflection of what on a national social and economic scale is discussed as the formation of 'organised capitalism'.

In order to make this heterogeneous mass of institutions and measures a little less cumbersome, they can be divided into four main types according to their function: regulation of the labour

---

(Göttingen, 1984), esp. pp. 220–40; G. Göckenjan, 'Medizin und Ärzte als Faktor der Disziplinierung der Unterschichten: Der Kassenarzt' in C. Sachsse and F. Tennstedt (eds), *Soziale Sicherheit und soziale Disziplinierung. Beiträge zu einer historischen Theorie der Sozialpolitik* (Frankfurt am Main, 1986), pp. 286–303; A. Labisch, '"Hygiene ist Moral — Moral ist Hygiene" — Soziale Disziplinierung durch Ärzte und Medizin' in Sachsse and Tennstedt, *Soziale Sicherheit*, pp. 265–85; idem, 'Doctors, Workers and the Scientific Cosmology of the Industrial World: The Social Construction of "Health" and the "Homo Hygienicus"', *Journal of Contemporary History*, 20(4) (1985); R.L. Schoenwald, 'Training Urban Man. A Hypothesis about the Sanitary Movement' in Dyos and Wolff, *The Victorian City*, pp. 669–92; F. Tennstedt, *Vom Proleten zum Industriearbeiter. Arbeiterbewegung und Sozialpolitik in Deutschland 1800 bis 1914* (Cologne, 1983), esp. pp. 448–70; P. Weindling, 'The Politics of Hygiene in Imperial Germany' in Labisch and Spree, *Medizin und sozialer Wandel*.

market (includes defining when someone is temporarily or in the longer term unfit for work); public health (divided into urban sanitation, standards of hygiene in housing and occupations); social welfare (divided between the largest problem groups such as mothers, infants, legitimate children, illegitimate children, consumptives, alcoholics and other outsiders); and population policy (encouraging parents to have larger families, discouraging contraception and abortion). It is also relevant to mention some important measures individually, such as compulsory inoculation for infants; binding public health regulations for water supply and particularly sewage disposal (introduction of WCs in towns); the catalogue of regulations laid out in the Sickness Insurance Act and social security legislation (official sanction given to doctors to decide on whether and why an individual is temporarily or permanently unfit for work; monopoly for doctors in defining the social role of the illness or the afflicted); measures on housing welfare; legally prescribed medical screening (for example, to establish fitness for military service, or in schools); medical tests in certain occupations (of those in public services, for example); state-sponsored campaigns to combat infant mortality, tuberculosis, alcoholism, and so on.

Beyond their immediate function, the social significance of these increasingly complementary measures and institutions resides in the fact that they forcibly introduced sections of the population to principles and forms of a rationalised life style, particularly those who hitherto had little experience of organising their lives in terms of time, economics and goals. At least as far as the measures detailed above were concerned, people were now going through this process every day in activities where attitudes to looking after one's body, health care, treating illnesses, family planning, birth and death played a crucial role. Consequently, the advance of these social and medical measures, together with the practical impact of the health-related infrastructure, meant that people were placed under enormous pressure to adapt and change their attitudes to these subjects. Social policy and infrastructural institutions did not merely create new life chances and redistribute some which were dependent on uncontrolled market forces, they also confronted the lower classes on a massive scale with what can be called the medical culture and its effective counterpart, a mechanistic view of the world.

There is no doubt that the most varied factors were at work in this process. The contribution made just by doctors, and the welfare campaign they greatly influenced and supported, can only

The Medicalisation of the Population

have been limited. Factory work, primary schools and, admittedly with some delay, military service were further institutions of 'enforced socialisation', inducing normal behaviour to be rationalised. Nevertheless one should not underestimate the effect that medical infrastructure and sickness insurance transmitted via organisations and institutions, although this did not take the form of a school learning process. The stimuli and pressures for adapting and changing values and behavioural patterns emanated from a kind of hidden curriculum established by the institutionalisation and bureaucratisation of the health service, the behavioural norms prevalent in the expanding medical infrastructure, and finally by social welfare measures and the Sickness Insurance Act.

It was not primarily consciousness and the intellect which were prey to its effects, but the daily activities which people performed and their related mentalities.[24] The sum of complementary demands and pressures on behaviour rendered the rationalisation of life style and the linked changes in values and mentalities an 'unconscious process'.[25] Since the aim of each of these demands and pressures was to produce an immediately perceptible result which in most cases the individual welcomed (preventing pain, keeping healthy, living longer, guaranteeing income levels, etc.), together they constituted an enforced learning process which must have had more chance of bringing about moral and practical change than one involving demands levelled at the individual's consciousness.

To this extent the contribution doctors made to long-term social change through the process of professionalisation can be regarded as relatively significant. They were the propagandists, executives and watchdogs of a whole range of the demands and pressures on everyday behaviour we have been discussing, in other words of the curriculum hidden in the infrastructure, in social security and in the welfare system. In this regard, their function was similar to that of the entrepreneurs and managers in the first factories who relied on factory rules, incentive schemes and specific forms of labour organisation. Alongside this function, which can be seen as deriving from the need to make the most profitable use of capital in production throughout the whole economy, from the point of view of a certain social elite — the propertied and educated bourgeoisie — such social measures and infrastructural institutions were intended

---

24. See P.R. Gleichmann, 'Die Verhäuslichung', pp. 261ff, 274ff.
25. See Imhof's introduction (cf. p. 176, n. 21), pp. 67–72; von Ferber, 'Gesellschaftliche Grundlagen', p. 3; idem, 'Volks- und Laienmedizin als Alternative zur wissenschaftlichen Medizin — Zur Partizipation im Gesundheitswesen', *Soziale Sicherheit*, 24 (1975), pp. 204–5.

to fulfil more specific functions. It is quite clear that these measures and institutions increasingly allowed representatives of the bourgeois elite to regiment, supervise and socialise the lower classes. Besides the desired effect of social integration, which, it must be said, was also welcomed by representatives of official policy at the end of the nineteenth century, there were further secondary aims which fully coincided with the ideological beliefs held by the propertied and educated bourgeoisie. These included: reducing infant mortality rates and improving fertility (preferably of married couples), in other words encouraging the growth of labour resources for military and productive purposes; inducing the working class to adapt their values and behaviour to bourgeois standards; neutralising the labour movement; and establishing 'racial hygiene' (*Rassenhygiene*).

The medicalisation of the lower classes, 'enforced socialisation' as we have called it, was already proceeding before the First World War, but in the 1920s it quickened pace. For doctors, it had important effects on professionalisation and on the growth in the market for their services. While it was still true in the late nineteenth century that with respect to geographical region and social strata 'the population exhibited greatly differing degrees of receptivity to increasingly professional and industrial medicine', this was gradually superseded in the early twentieth by 'homogenisation and standardisation which accompanied the growth of medical therapy. As conditions for this growth prospered in the wake of general economic expansion, the culture of medical science was able to take root in society'.[26] But this 'prescribed' medicalisation of the lower classes had even more far-reaching consequences. The market for the services offered by doctors had remained segmented up until the end of the nineteenth century, reflecting the existence of different subcultures, each with a distinct location, life style, value system, mentality and behavioural orientation. It would be dubious to contend that the population became 'homogenised' only in its receptivity to medical services. It is much more likely that these subcultural differences were ironed out at a deeper level and ultimately eradicated. At least in the long term, social homogenisation at the level of values, mentalities and behavioural orientations, that is of essential aspects of the life style of large sectors of the population, was more radical than would appear from the indicators which are normally used to describe structures of social inequality such as occupation, income, and level of education.

26. Von Ferber, *Soziologie*, p. 48.

Looked at in this way, the medicalisation of society, a process which to a considerable degree was initiated, carried through and supervised by doctors, and in particular the associated effect of the 'enforced socialisation of the lower classes', were important factors making for changes in the structures of social inequality in German society in the late nineteenth and early twentieth centuries. Social security and welfare and the medical infrastructure in particular redistributed the population's market-determined life chances to a certain extent, and, as health conditions for certain social and age groups were ameliorated, at the same time enabled people to try and improve their traditional market capacities in the long term through health care, family planning and better education (over a number of generations). The primary significance of these developments was that, despite the continued existence of clear inequalities in important 'components of market situation' (such as conditions at work and income levels), a process began by which values, mentalities and patterns of behaviour related to health were gradually made uniform throughout society. This was to have innumerable consequences because it affected important spheres of private reproduction (everyday life). Under the considerable pressure exerted by the medicalisation of society, values and mentalities began to reflect the way in which differences between subcultures and social strata were steadily being eroded, and tended less and less to correspond to the enduring class structure of society. The attempts by doctors to aid their own professionalisation by giving instrumental support to this levelling process and thus secure for themselves a privileged social position as an occupational group can be understood as an element in the dialectics of social change.

Conclusion

A résumé of my findings does not seem to be called for since the relevant conclusions to the various facets of the present study have already been set out in Sections 1.5, 2.5, 2.7, 3.3, and Chapters 6 and 11. My aim here is rather to suggest the significance that some aspects of my investigation have for the concept of social inequality developed in the introduction.

My basic premise is that class situation is the most important determinant of an individual's market capacity. Market capacity is understood as the totality of characteristics (both acquired and attributed), abilities and knowledge which command a value in the collective and individual exchange of life chances on the market. Consequently, a person's present or past social or occupational status also comes into play. As the early labour movement recognised, for the great mass of people who ever since the onset of industrialisation have not owned any means of production (i.e. the acquisition classes), health is a crucial component of market capacity. It is the most important factor affecting whether or not it is possible even to participate in the process of exchange, and determines to what extent one can attempt to improve a given market capacity by acquiring further components — for example by working overtime, undergoing further training (which is more important in the long run), or through political organisation. Not least, health is instrumental in deciding the occupational position and the related income level the individual may expect to reach, and for how long. Conversely, ill-health (in the form of acute and particularly chronic illnesses) limits market capacity to a greater or lesser degree.

By examining evidence of the varying incidence of illness and mortality rate according to age, sex, the size of the community (contrast between town and country), and occupational position, I have shown that there are class differences among dependent income-earners (blue- and white-collar workers and public officials). However, considerable changes took place during the period under investigation since almost all the social groups defined by these criteria were able to expand their market capacities as health improved in general. Blue-collar workers over the average

age of the working population, whose mortality rate dropped but whose health did not seem to improve to an equal degree, were the most important exception. In fact there is much evidence to suggest that a drop in the mortality rate of wage earners of both sexes in this age group was accompanied by rising morbidity, which manifested itself primarily as a cumulative deterioration of health and a gradual erosion of resistance to disease. Improvements in the health of children, young people and the young working population may have reduced somewhat the differences within the acquisition classes, perhaps even to the point where they became negligible. On the other hand, in the case of the older age groups of blue-collar workers of both sexes, class lines continued to be clearly, perhaps even more sharply defined, with working conditions impairing health and leading in this way to long-term collective social decline. Only a small number of these people will have been caught in the social security net established towards the end of the period we have studied here. Although the health of the other groups of dependent wage earners probably improved quite appreciably over this period, it is the resulting shifts in the patterns of disposable market capacities which are significant. On the basis of my evidence, in particular that relating to the social differences in infant mortality and death from tuberculosis, it can be concluded that, with respect to market capacities which depended upon and conversely affected health, blue-collar workers as a whole remained a deprived group even towards the end of the Empire period, while the position of public officials and white-collar workers in particular improved to a disproportionate degree, irrespective of the internal differences in these groups.

Several factors were involved in these changes in health and mortality. As we have seen, the expansion and improvement of the quality of medical services were of only secondary importance. By contrast it is highly likely that schemes to improve urban sanitation, which were very extensive by the end of the period under investigation, had a positive impact on the health of large sections of the urban population, with the larger towns benefiting at a much earlier stage than others. The introduction of a central water supply system, drainage, street cleaning and so on reduced the risks of infection and made everyday life more hygienic. Furthermore the emerging social security and welfare systems helped rationalise private reproduction (consumer behaviour, health care, domestic hygiene, etc.) and in the long term led to improvements in general health standards. As far as our period is concerned, however, it would appear that initially these social institutions — the infrastructure, social policy and social welfare — only served to exacerbate the health-dependent differences in market capacities, quite apart from the fact that large sections of the population remained beyond their reach. Where the persons involved did not have to show a positive interest, make a conscious effort or even show initiative in order to benefit from the measures and institutions, they tended to equalise opportunities. (A good example was the way in which the incidence of typhoid in Berlin fell on average and no longer varied with social class after the introduction of a central water supply system.) Where, however, the individual needed to show some initiative in order to take advantage of the expanding health sector, infrastructure and in particular the welfare services and advisory schemes, it was on the whole the lower and middle strata of the middle classes, i.e. the majority of the 'new middle class', who initially benefited. The typical demands placed on these social groups in their occupational settings endowed them with the necessary information and skills required to deal with the bureaucracy and apply the rules of rational behaviour. In contrast, for the lower classes, this information was an absolute prerequisite and, for them to obtain it, certain traditional social barriers had to be broken down. The 'enforced socialisation' brought about by social security and welfare systems played some part here. But this primarily set in motion a longer-term process of social learning which in particular transformed mentalities and patterns of typical behaviour and which was to last over two generations. This explains why the social differences in market capacities which depended on health became as acute as they did between the rural and urban lower strata, on the one hand, and within the latter, on the other, with skilled/unskilled and organised/unorganised generally forming the dividing lines. Those with fixed employment, especially skilled workers, came to take up positions in the class structure increasingly similar to those occupied by middle and junior public officials and white-collar workers, while the great mass of unskilled labourers were clearly left behind.

Differentiation by class is augmented and to an extent modified by social stratification. By the latter I mean not only the attribution of different values and the maintenance of corresponding social relationships in the sense of 'differential association'. As far as I am concerned, an essential element of stratification is that it also expresses a particular mode of living and the mentalities related to it. To a degree, certain patterns of values and behaviour are also involved here. It can thus be understood why stratification is not an absolute and linear function of class structure and does not coincide with it completely in terms of social differentiation. By examining the relationship between nutrition methods and infant mortality, I was able to demonstrate, for example, that the effect of certain feeding habits was either to strengthen the impact of market capacity on health, or clearly weaken it, if not even cancel it out entirely. The effects which being a member of the labour movement had on the market capacity of workers must also be considered here. In the medium and long term, members became more enlightened and more aware and were probably able to increase their market capacity. It cannot be doubted that the labour movement contributed to the medicalisation of the lower strata. As an element in social stratification, participation in the class-orientated labour movement added to the gradual levelling out of class differences in those market capacities dependent on health.

As far as structures of social inequality are concerned, my investigation shows the following trends. Among the acquisition classes, health standards did generally improve up to the end of the period studied, and these components of market capacity on the whole became more valuable. But at the same time the differences between groups within classes grew. On the other hand, the long-term effect of some elements in social stratification was to make health standards more uniform throughout society — here the medicalisation of the population, particularly of the lower strata, can be seen as a process by which values, mentalities and patterns of behaviour relating to health became standardised. This process, which involved the most varied factors and groups, led to a situation where structures of social inequality were gradually reflected less and less at the level of values and mentalities. With regard to the types of values and mentalities which shape behaviour during illness and reproductive behaviour, particularly attitudes to the body and health, it is much more appropriate to say that differences to be found between specific subcultures and strata progressively levelled off during the first half of the twentieth century. Increasingly, it is in society's peripheral groups that one finds considerable differences, and even there market capacities are not ultimately dependent upon such factors. Thus although various indicators show that where illness and mortality are concerned, social inequality increased during the period I have been examining, there are also a number of factors suggesting that, in the longer term (particularly after the First World War), differences in health and mortality were increasingly reduced, with the consequence that market capacities determined by health became more evenly distributed throughout society.

Appendix

Table 1: Mortality rates in various age groups and regions in Prussia in 1876, 1901, 1913 (per 10,000 in each age group)

Year	Age group	Pr	Kö	Gu	Ar	Dü	Be	Do	Es	Fr
1876	0–1	2055	2181	2207	1512	1680	2950	1883	2015	1652
	>1–15	168	190	185	207	185	257	244	240	166
	>15–30	66	58	64	81	80	68	88	75	66
	>30–60	150	164	172	167	164	155	197	178	161
	>60–70	481	520	512	535	494	463	565	490	541
	All groups	256	269	275	254	252	301	290	285	208
1901	0–1	1997	2185	2496	1590	1678	2243	1907	1631	1547
	>1–15	104	127	151	127	113	104	129	178	81
	>15–30	50	49	54	56	49	46	48	48	44
	>30–60	117	115	111	125	115	122	136	127	126
	>60–70	411	376	370	466	434	410	452	516	446
	All groups	207	227	252	199	190	180	204	213	158
1913	0–1	1420	1853	1951	1255	1216	.	.	.	.
	>1–15	58	60	60	67	54	.	.	.	.
	>15–30	41	42	39	47	41	.	.	.	.
	>30–60	94	103	95	95	87	.	.	.	.
	>60–70	380	353	347	420	398	.	.	.	.
	All groups	149	177	182	137	125	140	.	.	.

Key: Pr = Kingdom of Prussia; Kö = Administrative District (AD) of Königsberg; Gu = AD of Gumbinnen; Ar = AD of Arnsberg; Dü = AD of Düsseldorf; Be = Berlin; Do = Dortmund; Es = Essen; Fr = Frankfurt am Main.

Sources: Calculated from *Preußische Statistik*, vols. 46, 179, 189; *Das Gesundheitswesen des preußischen Staates in Jahre* ... (for 1903 and 1913); *Medizinal-statistische Mitteilungen aus dem Kaiserlichen Gesundheitsamte*, vol. 19 (Berlin, 1917).

Table 2: Mortality rates[1] in various age groups in 22 large Prussian towns[2] and in the state of Prussia as a whole in 1876 and 1900 (number of deaths during the year per 10,000 of the age group alive on 1 January)

	0–1	1–2	2–3	3–5	5–10	10–15	15–20	20–25	25–30	30–40	40–50	50–60	60–70	70–80	80+	All groups	All groups except 0–1
								1876									
22 large Prussian towns	3272	920	471	265	106	33	56	75	104	153	248	360	629	1138	2288	300	187
Prussia (average)	2739	732	360	219	88	38	53	80	85	108	166	269	521	1082	2261	275	187
								1900									
22 large Prussian towns	2938	623	218	121	52	28	38	49	59	85	139	243	493	1031	2189	213	137
Prussia (average)	2582	529	199	115	50	31	39	56	61	78	123	209	479	1001	2607	223	149

[1] Figures for 1876 refer to males only.
[2] Towns with population over 100,000 in 1900.

Sources: Calculated from *Preußische Statistik*, vol. 46, (Berlin, 1878), pp. xviii, xx–xxi, 156–7; *Das Sanitätswesen des preußischen Staates während der Jahre 1898, 1899 und 1900* (Berlin, 1903), pp. 9 and 16–21; *Preußische Statistik*, vol. 171 (Berlin, 1902), p. 20.

Appendix

Table 3: Correlation[1] between infant mortality rate[2] and welfare,[3] and excess mortality rates[4] in urban districts of Berlin[5] from 1886 to 1910

Indicator	1886	1900	1910
Product moment correlation coefficient	–0.91	–0.73	–0.82
Maximum infant mortality figure per 1000 (district)	381 (Wedding)	313 (Königsviertel)	239 (Gesundbrunnen)
Minimum infant mortality figure per 1000 (district)	202 (Friedrichstadt)	138 (Friedrichstadt)	112 (Friedrichstadt)
Excess mortality rate (%)	89	127	113

1. Measured using product moment correlation of infant mortality with welfare index per district.
2. Infant mortality rates refers to number of infant per 1000 who died during first year (includes legitimate and illegitimate offspring, and still-births).
3. Welfare index is the figure obtained by dividing the average rent in the district by the number of inhabitants per room using figures for 1910.
4. Excess mortality rate calculated as a percentage ratio of maximum to minimum infant mortality rate.
5. Districts until 1910 are the 15 Registry Offices in Old Berlin listed for 1886 (excluding VI = Luisenstadt city side of the canal including Neukölln because mortality rates in children's home there entirely distort the figures). Births and deaths in institutions and hospitals are included in the data for the parental district of residence.

Sources: Calculated from Statistisches Amt der Stadt Berlin (eds), *Die Grundstücks-Aufnahme vom 15. Okt. 1910 sowie die Wohnungs- und Bevölkerungs-Aufnahme vom 1. Dez. 1910 in der Stadt Berlin* (Berlin, 1914), section 1, no. 2, pp. 2ff. and 50–5; *Statistisches Jahrbuch der Stadt Berlin*, vol. 14 (1886–7), p. 62; vol. 27 (1900–2), p. 92; vol. 32 (1908–11), p. 133.

Table 4: Infant mortality rates in different occupational groups[1] in Prussia from 1877 to 1913. (Percentage average for two- and three-year periods, incl. illegitimate children, excl. still-births. Groups determined by occupation of father for legitimate and of mother for illegitimate children.)

Occupational groups	1877–9	1880–2	1883–5	1886–8	1889–91	1892–3	1894–5	1896–7	1898–9	1900–1	1902–3	1904–5	1906–7	1908–9	1910–11	1912–13
Self-employed	18.2	18.4	18.7	18.3	18.3	18.3	17.6	17.0	17.1	17.6	16.0	16.3	14.6	14.3	14.5	12.3
Public officials	17.5	18.0	17.8	17.0	16.3	16.2	15.6	14.9	14.7	15.3	12.5	12.9	11.0	10.0	9.9	8.3
White-collar	18.6	18.1	18.3	18.0	17.3	17.4	17.1	16.1	16.1	16.6	13.6	13.7	12.0	10.9	11.6	9.3
'Skilled' workers	18.9	19.8	20.2	19.7	19.6	19.9	19.3	18.7	19.0	19.4	17.1	18.1	16.2	15.4	15.9	13.1
'Unskilled' workers	20.6	21.6	22.3	21.8	22.2	22.8	22.6	22.5	22.2	23.7	20.2	21.7	19.7	19.4	20.0	17.4
Domestics, household servants	29.6	29.9	30.5	21.5	29.9	30.0	29.7	28.5	28.6	31.0	26.6	28.2	25.5	25.2	25.8	22.5
Total population	20.1	20.8	21.2	20.6	20.6	20.9	20.4	19.8	19.9	20.6	18.3	19.1	17.3	16.8	17.2	14.8

1. Up to 1901 armed forces excluded. From 1902 groups composed as follows (symbols taken from *Preußische Statistik*): self-employed = Aa, Ab, Ba, Ca (up to 1901 incl. liberal professions); public officials = Ea, Eb, Ec (after 1901 incl. liberal professions and armed forces); white-collar = Bb, Cb; 'skilled' workers = Bc, Cc, Cd; 'unskilled' workers = Ad, Bd, D2; domestics and household servants = Ac,D1.

Sources: K. Seutemann, *Kindersterblichkeit*, Appendix, table XIV (up to 1888); I have recalculated Seutemann's figures by subtracting still-births; after 1888 from *Preußische Statistik*, vols. 113, 117, 123, 127, 134, 138, 143, 149, 155, 160, 164, 169, 178, 183, 190, 196, 200, 207, 213, 220, 224, 229, 233, 238, and 245.

Appendix

Table 5: Excess infant mortality rates in different occupational groups compared with public officials and (after 1902) the liberal professions in Prussia from 1877 to 1913 (percentages, excl. stillbirths)

Occupational group	1877	1886	1895	1900	1905	1910	1913
White-collar	6	7	12	12	1	11	12
Self-employed	4	6	11	16	27	45	53
'Skilled' workers	8	14	25	29	37	52	64
'Unskilled' workers	17	25	44	56	71	97	119
Domestics/servants	67	71	92	104	126	158	183
Average for total population	15	19	30	37	49	69	85

Sources: As Table 4.

Table 6: Infant mortality rates in different occupational groups in Prussia from 1902 to 1913. Group determined by occupation of father for legitimate and of mother for illegitimate offspring (average percentage over two-year period, excl. still-births)

Occupational group		1902–3	1904–5	1906–7	1908–9	1910–11	1912–13	Decline (%) from 1902–3 to 1912–13
Self-employed	Agriculture	15.8	15.9	14.6	14.7	14.7	12.9	18
	Manufacturing/craft	16.3	16.6	14.7	14.1	14.4	11.9	27
	Trade/commerce	16.1	16.5	14.4	13.5	13.7	10.9	32
Public officials	Senior officials and lib. profs.	11.0	11.0	9.5	8.5	8.2	6.9	37
	Junior officials	13.8	14.4	12.3	11.1	11.3	9.5	31
White-collar	Manufacturing/craft	14.1	14.0	12.3	11.3	11.9	9.4	33
	Trade/commerce	12.9	13.2	11.6	10.4	11.0	9.1	29
'Skilled' workers	Manufacturing/craft	17.2	18.2	16.4	15.6	16.2	13.4	22
	Trade/commerce	16.6	17.5	15.4	14.6	15.1	12.4	25
'Unskilled' workers	Agriculture	20.4	21.6	20.0	20.7	21.0	19.1	6
	Manufacturing/craft	20.0	21.7	19.5	18.7	19.4	16.4	18
Domestic/servants		26.6	28.2	25.5	25.2	25.8	22.5	15
Total population		18.3	19.1	17.3	16.8	17.2	14.8	19

Source: Preußische Statistik, vols. 183, 190, 196, 200, 207, 213, 220, 224, 229, 233, 238, 245.

Table 7: Percentage of legitimate infants[1] breast-fed in various income groups in selected towns (T) and rural districts (D) of western Germany from 1905 to 1911[2]

Father's taxable annual income (Marks)	Barmen (T) 1905	Essen (T) 1908	Geldern (D) 1910	Grevenbroich (D) 1911	Mönchengladbach (T) 1909	Moers (D) 1910	Neuss (D) 1908	Rheydt (T) 1909	Average percentage breast-fed (excl. Barmen)[3]	Average percentage breast-fed (excl. Essen[4] and Barmen)
1	2	3	4	5	6	7	8	9	10	11
up to 900	81	76	79	72	56	74	63	61	73(n=1802)	72(n=1379)
901–1500	69	80	76	70	62	70	67	65	72(n=8536)	68(n=5228)
1501–3000		78	66	56	52	68	66	58	71(n=3984)	64(n=1687)
3000+	48	59	44	33	49	41	35	38	49(n=362)	41(n=172)

1. Infants = children aged up to 1 year   2. In each income group all other infants were not fed with mother's milk   3. Incomplete data   4. High absolute figures dominate average.

Sources:

Column 2: Kriege and Seutemann, 'Ernährungsverhältnisse und Sterblichkeit der Säuglinge in Barmen', *Centralblatt für allgemeine Gesundheitspflege*, 25 (1906), p. 22.

Column 3: H. Lübbering, 'Die Sterblichkeit der Säuglinge in Essen mit besonderer Berücksichtigung ihrer Ernährungsweise', *Zeitschrift für Säuglingsfürsorge*, 6 (1912), pp. 354ff.

Column 4: M. Baum, 'Lebensbedingungen und Sterblichkeit der Säuglinge in den Kreisen Moers und Geldern', *Zeitschrift für Säuglingsfürsorge*, 4 (1911), p. 319.

Column 5: M. Baum, 'Lebensbedingungen und Sterblichkeit der Säuglinge im Kreise Grevenbroich', *Zeitschrift für Säuglingsfürsorge*, 6 (1912), p. 207.

Column 6: M. Baum, 'Sterblichkeit und Lebensbedingungen der Säuglinge in den Stadtkreisen M.-Gladbach und Rheydt und in dem Landkreise M.-Gladbach', *Zeitschrift für soziale Medizin*, 5 (1910), p. 86.

Column 7: As for column 4, p. 320.

Column 8: M. Baum, 'Sterblichkeit und Lebensbedingungen der Säuglinge im Kreise Neuß', *Zeitschrift für soziale Medizin*, 4 (1909), p. 513.

Column 9: As for column 6, p. 87.

Appendix

Table 8: Breast-feeding and mortality of legitimate infants in various income groups in the administrative district of Düsseldorf from 1905 to 1911. (For every 100 living, legitimate infants (aged up to 12 months), divided according to feeding method and income group, the number of infants who died during their first year was as shown.)

Region (date)	Breast-fed children Father's income (Marks)		Children not breast-fed Father's income (Marks)	
	≤1500	>1500	≤1500	>1500
Towns				
Barmen (1905)	7.3	6.4	31.6	12.5
Mönchengladbach (1909)	9.6	7.3	23.4	13.5
Neuß (1908)	12.2	5.8	43.2	20.2
Rheydt (1909)	7.1	5.7	20.5	11.3
Rural districts				
Geldern (1910)	6.3	3.3	16.7	5.7
Gladbach (1909)	9.5	8.5	29.7	19.2
Grevenbroich (1911)	9.9	8.7	42.1	23.6
Moers (1910)	7.4	4.8	19.7	18.7
Neuß (excl. town, 1908)	9.2	4.9	28.2	19.6
Average	8.7	6.2	28.3	16.0

Source: M. Baum, 'Lebensbedingungen und Sterblichkeit der Säuglinge im Kreise Grevenbroich', *Zeitschrift für Säuglingsfürsorge*, 6 (6) (1912), p. 313.

Table 9: Breast-feeding and mortality of legitimate children in various income groups in Hanover and Linden in 1911–12. (For every 100 living, legitimate infants (aged up to 12 months) divided according to feeding method and income group, the number of infants who died in their first year was as shown.)

Region	Breast-fed children Father's income (Marks)		Children not breast-fed Father's income (Marks)	
	≤1800	>1800	≤1800	>1800
Hanover	9.6	5.8	27.3	11.2
Linden (near Hanover)	9.5	7.5	36.0	18.9

Source: Komitee zur Ermittlung der Säuglingsernährung in Hannover-Linden (eds), *Säuglingsernährung, Säuglingssterblichkeit und Säuglingsschutz in den Städten Hannover und Linden* (Berlin, 1913), pp. 69, 94.

Appendix

Table 10: Breast-feeding, legitimacy and mother's employment in Hanover in 1912. (For the 740 infants living with their mothers[1] on 4 June 1912 in Hanover, the table shows the mother's occupation[2] and whether she breast-fed her child.)

Type of occupation	%	legitimate of which % breast-fed	%	illegitimate of which % breast-fed
Occupation at home				
Assistant in husband's trade/business	28	52	–	–
Self-employed tradeswoman	3	29	–	–
Tailoress, seamstress	8	50	11	38
Washerwoman, ironer	2	73	–	–
Milliner, embroiderer	1	70	1	100
Others	3	58	4	60
Average percentage of infants breast-fed by mothers working at home		52		48
Occupation outside home				
Waitress, washerwoman, cleaner	28	48	17	21
Delivery girl	3	44	–	–
Tradeswoman	2	23	–	–
Tailoress, seamstress, hairdresser, etc.	1	25	6	11
Commercial white-collar	1	33	9	17
Factory worker	19	29	48	19
Others	1	33	4	40
Average number of infants breast-fed by mothers working outside home		39		20
Total	100% (=600)		100% (=140)	

1. Data on a total of 5,086 infants in Hanover were collected. Of these, 1,026

Appendix

(approx. 20%) had mothers who worked. This average is greatly distorted, however, since in only 661 cases of the legitimate infants (approx. 15%) did the mothers work, while this figure was 365 (approx. 64%) for illegitimate infants. Only cases where the infant lived with the mother are included in the table. Thus 61 (approx. 9%) working mothers of legitimate infants and 225 (approx. 62%) working mothers of illegitimate infants are excluded. Consequently the table offers no conclusive evidence about the distribution of occupations among unmarried mothers since only a fraction of these are included.

2. Some occupational groups are so underrepresented (as can be tested by recalculating percentages) that the corresponding figures on breast-feeding are unrepresentative.

Source: Komitee zur Ermittlung der Säuglingsernährung in Hannover-Linden (eds), *Säuglingsernährung, Säuglingssterblichkeit und Säuglingsschutz in den Städten Hannover und Linden* (Berlin, 1913), pp. 52–4.

Table 11: Duration of breast-feeding[1] of legitimate infants[2] in selected areas of north-west Germany in different income groups from 1905 to 1912

Key: n = number of infants   B = percentage of those who were breast-fed

Duration of breast-feeding (months)	Barmen 1905				Admin. district of Düsseldorf[3] 1908–11				Hanover and Linden 1912			
	≤1500[4]		>1500[4]		≤1500[4]		>1500[4]		≤1500[4]		>1500[4]	
	n	B	n	B	n	B	n	B	n	B	n	B
1	2	3	4	5	6	7	8	9	10	11	12	13
≤3	931	91	129	90	3482	84	924	80	1375	81	300	82
3–6	916	84	144	67	3166	70	858	63	1206	56	265	54
6–9	831	76	135	51	3111	62	820	53	1178	45	222	33
9–12	805	70	160	48	2958	54	833	41	1189	36	237	22

1. Duration of breast-feeding calculated as proportion of breast-fed infants in each age and income group.
2. Children up to age of 12 months.
3. Weighted averages from data for the districts of Geldern, Grevenbroich, Mönchen-Gladbach, Moers and Neuß and for the town of Rheydt. Düsseldorf itself is not included. Otherwise the averages can safely be taken as representative for the administrative district.
4. Father's taxable annual income (Marks).

Source: Calculated from sources cited for Tables 7 and 12.

Table 12: Duration of breast-feeding of legitimate infants living with their mothers on 4 June 1912 in Hanover (Hanover and Linden)[1] in different occupational groups
Key: n = number of infants   B = percentage of those who were breast-fed

Father's occupation	Academics: all types		Middle public officials + non-graduate teachers		Self-employed		White-collar		Junior public officials + NCOs		Labourers + factory workers	
Age of infant (months)	n	B	n	B	n	B	n	B	n	B	n	B
≤3	46	85	44	82	170	81	158	80	78	80	1092	81
3–6	43	44	30	60	174	53	143	53	52	64	939	57
6–9	40	33	29	41	143	32	98	35	86	56	916	45
9–12	38	16	46	28	144	26	119	19	77	31	941	38

1. Since Linden was, so to speak, 'purely' a workers' quarter, representation of other social groups is sufficiently low to be excluded.

Source: Calculated from Komitee zur Ermittlung der Säuglingsernährung in Hannover-Linden (eds), *Säuglingsernährung, Säuglingssterblichkeit und Säuglingsschutz in den Städten Hannover und Linden*, (Berlin, 1913), pp. 54–5, 81–2.

Appendix

Table 13: Average number of children per complete marriage[1] in various social groups in Lower Saxony[2] from the end of eighteenth century to 1914

Date of marriage	'New middle class' Educated strata[3]	Upwardly mobile strata[4]	Total	Self-employed in trade and commerce	Farmers[5]
before 1800	5.8	–	5.7	–	6.7
1800–49	5.8	–	5.5	–	6.2
1850–74	4.3	–	4.2	4.4	5.4
1875–99	2.9	3.4	3.1	4.3	4.2
1900–14	2.5	2.6	2.5	2.8	3.5

1. Complete marriage = woman married before age of 30 and marriage lasted at least until woman's 45th year (i.e. end of child-bearing period).
2. Figures are based on 49 geneaologies of middle-class and farming families (some 3000 individual families) in Lower Saxony. More exact details of geographical area are not given.
3. The 'new middle class' includes all public officials, white-collar workers and graduates in the liberal professions. The educated strata includes senior administrative and judicial officials, diplomats and senior political functionaries, military officers from lieutenant upwards, university teachers and secondary school teachers, and the liberal professions (excluding engineers and architects).
4. Senior employees in the economy including engineers and architects, middle and junior public officials including non-graduate teachers, middle-level and junior state and private white-collar workers.
5. Owners of large and medium-size farms, and tenants with or without rights of inheritance.

Source: A. von Nell, 'Die Entwicklung der generativen Strukturen bürgerlicher and bäuerlicher Familien von 1750 bis zur Gegenwart' (unpubl. diss., Bochum, 1973), pp. 29, 58, 94.

Appendix

Table 14: Average number of children per marriage[1] in the German Reich[2] by occupation[3], economic sector and year of marriage, in the late nineteenth and early twentieth centuries

Occupational group	Year of marriage					
	pre-1905	1905–9	1910–14	1915–19	1920–24	1925–29
Agricultural						
Self-employed	5.5	4.6	4.1	3.5	3.1	2.7
Workers	6.1	5.2	4.7	4.1	3.5	3.0
Agric. pop. in total	5.5	4.7	4.1	3.6	3.2	2.8
Non-agricultural						
Self-employed	4.0	3.1	2.6	2.2	1.9	1.7
Public officials and professional soldiers	3.5	2.9	2.5	2.1	1.8	1.6
Non-manual workers	3.4	2.7	2.3	1.9	1.6	1.5
Manual workers	4.7	3.8	3.3	2.8	2.4	2.1
Non-agric. pop. in total	4.5	3.4	2.9	2.4	2.1	1.9
Total average	4.7	3.6	3.1	2.6	2.3	2.0

1. Figures are based on all first marriages (including childless couples) as of May 1939, and include all legitimate, legitimated ante-nuptial and deceased children, still-births, children living away from home, and offspring of separated parents.
2. German Reich of May 1939 (excluding Memelland, but including Austria).
3. Data were collected on the husband's occupation, occupational position, and branch and sector of the economy.

Source: Calculated from *Volkszählung. Die Familien im Deutschen Reich*, compiled by the Statistical Office of the Reich (Berlin, 1943) ('Volks- Berufs- und Betriebszählung vom 17.5.1939', *Statistik des Deutschen Reichs*, vol. 554), pp. 62–81.

Appendix

Table 15: Average number of children per marriage in the non-agricultural population of the German Reich, by occupation, size of community and year of marriage, late nineteenth and early twentieth centuries. Table shows absolute numbers and (in brackets) the figure as a percentage of the average number of children for the group in all communities.

Occupational group	pre-1905	1905–9	1910–14	1915–19	1920–24	1925–29
Communities with less than 2,000 inhabitants						
Self-employed	4.9	4.0	3.4	2.9	2.5	2.2
	(121)	(128)	(131)	(132)	(131)	(130)
Public officials and professional soldiers	4.3	3.7	3.2	2.7	2.3	2.0
	(123)	(126)	(127)	(126)	(127)	(124)
White-collar	4.3	3.6	3.1	2.6	2.3	2.0
	(127)	(134)	(138)	(137)	(140)	(137)
Blue-collar	5.4	4.6	4.0	3.5	3.0	2.5
	(115)	(121)	(124)	(127)	(126)	(124)
Communities with between 2,000 and 100,000 inhabitants						
Self-employed	4.2	3.2	2.7	2.3	2.0	1.7
	(103)	(104)	(104)	(105)	(103)	(103)
Public officials and professional soldiers	3.8	3.2	2.7	2.3	2.0	1.8
	(108)	(108)	(108)	(108)	(109)	(109)
White-collar	3.7	2.9	2.5	2.1	1.8	1.6
	(109)	(111)	(111)	(112)	(112)	(112)
Blue-collar	4.9	4.1	3.5	2.9	2.5	2.1
	(105)	(106)	(107)	(105)	(104)	(104)
Communities with at least 200,000 inhabitants						
Self-employed	3.2	2.3	1.9	1.6	1.3	1.1
	(79)	(74)	(73)	(71)	(68)	(68)
Public officials and professional soldiers	3.0	2.4	2.1	1.8	1.4	1.3
	(84)	(83)	(82)	(82)	(79)	(80)
White-collar	2.9	2.2	1.9	1.6	1.3	1.2
	(86)	(84)	(83)	(83)	(81)	(82)
Blue-collar	3.9	3.1	2.6	2.1	1.8	1.6
	(84)	(80)	(78)	(76)	(74)	(76)

Source: As Table 14.

Table 16: Average number of children per marriage in the German Reich, by 43 occupations and year of marriage, late nineteenth and early twentieth centuries

Occupational group	Number of children Year of marriage						Group's rank Year of marriage					
	Before 1905 (1)	1905–09 (2)	1910–14 (3)	1915–19 (4)	1920–24 (5)	1925–29 (6)	Before 1905 (1)	1905–09 (2)	1910–14 (3)	1915–19 (4)	1920–24 (5)	1925–29 (6)
Agriculture												
Self-employed peasants, gardeners, fishermen, etc.	5.6	4.7	4.1	3.5	3.1	2.7	41	41	41	42	42	41
Blue-collar workers in agriculture etc.	6.0	5.2	4.7	4.1	3.5	3.0	43	43	43	43	43	43
Self-employed												
Self-employed artisans and craftsmen	4.4	3.5	2.9	2.4	2.2	1.9	32	31	31	30	32	28
Self-employed in other industrial occupations and crafts	3.8	3.0	2.5	2.1	1.8	1.7	24	23	23	18	18	17
Self-employed in trade	3.6	2.7	2.3	1.9	1.7	1.5	22	20	16	13	11	7
Self-employed in transport	4.4	3.3	2.7	2.3	2.0	1.8	31	27	26	26	26	24
Self-employed in hotels and catering	4.0	3.0	2.5	2.0	1.8	1.5	26	24	22	15	16	8
Self-employed doctors	2.6	2.5	2.3	2.1	2.0	2.0	4	15	15	16	24	31
Self-employed apothecaries	2.7	2.3	2.1	1.7	1.5	1.6	6	4	5	3	5	13
Self-employed writers, freelance scholars, etc.	2.8	2.0	1.8	1.4	1.3	1.1	10	1	1	1	1	1
Self-employed artists, actors, etc.	3.1	2.3	2.0	1.5	1.4	1.1	15	3	3	2	2	2
Self-employed lawyers and notaries	3.0	2.4	2.2	1.9	1.8	1.7	12	12	14	12	14	20
Public officials and all holding official status												
Army and navy officers, etc.	2.1	2.3	2.1	1.9	1.7	1.6	1	6	8	11	13	16
Army NCOs, etc.	2.7	2.4	2.2	2.2	1.9	1.8	5	9	12	25	20	23
Church officials	3.9	3.4	3.3	2.9	2.7	2.7	25	30	36	38	38	42

Train drivers, guards, etc.	4.3	3.6	3.1	2.5	2.1	1.6	30	34	33	31	29	15		
Other officials of Imperial Post Office and Railways	3.5	2.9	2.5	2.2	1.9	1.6	21	22	24	24	19	11		
Doctors	2.7	2.4	2.3	2.1	2.0	2.0	7	10	17	19	23	32		
University rectors and lecturers	2.7	2.6	2.4	2.2	1.9	1.9	8	18	19	22	21	30		
Senior secondary school teachers and headmasters	2.5	2.3	2.2	2.0	1.8	1.7	3	7	10	14	15	19		
Primary school teachers, etc.	3.0	2.7	2.4	2.1	1.9	1.9	14	19	20	21	22	27		
Judges, lawyers junior barristers	2.5	2.4	2.1	1.9	1.7	1.7	2	14	7	8	9	18		
Police officers etc.	3.2	2.3	2.2	1.9	1.7	1.6	18	2	13	7	10	14		
Policemen	3.2	2.8	2.4	2.1	1.7	1.5	19	21	21	17	12	9		
Other officials (mainly in admin. and bureaucracy)	3.2	2.5	2.2	1.9	1.6	1.6	16	16	9	10	8	12		
White-collar workers														
Salaried doctors	2.8	2.4	2.3	2.2	2.1	2.0	9	11	18	23	28	35		
Book-keepers, others in financial administration, etc.	3.0	2.3	2.0	1.7	1.5	1.3	13	8	2	4	3	4		
Other senior white-collar workers	2.9	2.3	2.0	1.8	1.5	1.5	11	5	4	5	6	6		
White-collar foremen	3.8	3.0	2.6	2.1	1.8	1.6	23	25	25	20	17	10		
Other white-collar (mainly admin. and bureaucracy)	3.3	2.6	2.2	1.9	1.6	1.4	20	17	11	9	7	5		
Blue-collar workers														
Miners and others in mining industry	5.7	4.9	4.1	3.3	2.9	2.4	42	42	42	41	40	38		
Workers in stone, glass and ceramics industries	5.4	4.5	3.9	3.3	2.8	2.4	40	40	40	40	39	39		
Workers in ferrous industries	4.3	3.4	2.9	2.4	2.1	1.8	29	29	29	27	27	22		
Chemical workers	4.8	3.9	3.3	2.9	2.5	2.1	38	38	38	37	37	37		
Textile workers	4.5	3.7	3.2	2.6	2.2	1.8	34	35	35	33	31	25		

continued on p. 208

Table 16: *continued*

	(1)	(2)	(3)	(4)	(5)	(6)	(1)	(2)	(3)	(4)	(5)	(6)
Workers in paper industry	4.7	3.9	3.3	2.8	2.4	2.0	37	37	37	36	36	36
Workers in printing industry	3.2	2.4	2.1	1.8	1.5	1.3	17	13	6	6	4	3
Workers in tanning and leather goods industries	4.2	3.4	2.9	2.4	2.1	1.9	28	28	28	29	30	26
Workers in woodworking, carving and toy industries	4.5	3.5	3.0	2.7	2.3	2.0	33	32	32	34	34	34
Workers in food industry	4.6	3.6	3.0	2.6	2.2	1.9	36	33	31	32	33	29
Workers in clothing industry	4.1	3.2	2.8	2.4	2.0	1.7	27	26	27	28	25	21
Construction workers	5.2	4.4	3.8	3.3	2.9	2.4	39	39	39	39	41	40
Other blue-collar (incl. domestic helps)	4.6	3.7	3.2	2.7	2.3	2.0	35	36	34	35	35	33
All co-habiting married couples	4.7	3.6	3.1	2.6	2.3	2.0						

Source: As Table 14.

Table 17: Distribution of married couples in each occupational group by number of children and year of marriage (per cent)

Occupational group	Marriage before 1905 number of children						Marriage 1905–09 number of children					
	0	1	2	3	4	5+	0	1	2	3	4	5+
Agriculture												
Self-employed peasants, gardeners, fishermen, etc.	4	6	10	11	12	57	5	7	13	15	14	46
Blue-collar workers in agriculture, etc.	4	5	7	9	11	63	5	7	11	12	13	53
Self-employed												
Self-employed artisans and craftsmen	6	9	15	16	14	41	7	13	20	18	14	27
Self-employed in other industrial occupations and crafts	7	11	18	18	15	32	9	16	24	19	12	19
Self-employed in trade	9	12	19	17	13	30	12	19	24	18	11	16
Self-employed in transport	7	9	14	15	13	41	10	15	21	18	13	24
Self-employed in hotels and catering	7	10	16	16	14	35	10	15	22	19	13	20
Self-employed doctors	11	13	27	23	13	13	13	14	27	22	13	10
Self-employed apothecaries	9	14	29	23	13	13	12	19	29	22	11	8
Self-employed writers, freelance scholars, etc.	14	15	22	20	10	19	25	21	19	18	9	9
Self-employed artists, actors, etc.	13	16	19	17	13	22	20	23	22	13	10	12
Self-employed lawyers and notaries	9	12	21	24	16	17	13	15	27	23	13	9
Public officials and all holding official status												
Army and navy officers, etc.	13	24	24	25	7	7	14	15	31	21	12	8
Army NCOs, etc.	28	23	15	7	8	19	16	22	20	18	11	13
Church officials	9	7	14	18	16	35	9	8	18	22	16	27
Train drivers, guards, etc.	4	8	15	17	16	40	5	12	21	19	15	28

continued on p. 210

Table 17: *continued*

	0	1	2	3	4	5+	0	1	2	3	4	5+
Other officials of Imperial Post Office and Railways	6	13	21	19	14	26	7	18	25	20	12	18
Doctors	14	15	23	24	8	16	11	18	26	23	15	7
University rectors and lecturers	14	11	24	20	16	16	12	10	27	24	16	10
Senior secondary school teachers and headmasters	8	17	35	19	9	11	11	19	29	22	10	8
Primary school teachers, etc.	5	16	26	21	13	18	7	20	29	20	11	13
Judges, lawyers, junior barristers	18	11	26	20	12	14	9	17	30	22	13	9
Police officers, etc.	22	11	17	22	0	28	14	19	28	23	7	9
Policemen	9	15	21	18	12	24	7	19	27	19	14	15
Other officials (mainly in admin. and bureaucracy)	7	15	23	19	14	22	9	21	28	19	10	12
White-collar workers												
Salaried doctors	12	10	19	27	19	14	15	18	25	18	15	11
Book-keepers, others in financial administration etc.	9	17	23	18	12	20	12	23	27	17	10	11
Other senior white-collar workers	11	16	24	19	13	17	12	22	28	18	10	10
White-collar foremen	6	11	18	18	15	32	8	17	24	19	13	20
Other white-collar (mainly admin. and bureaucracy)	10	15	20	17	13	25	12	21	26	18	11	14
Blue-collar workers												
Miners and others in mining industry	5	6	9	9	12	60	4	6	12	14	15	49
Workers in stone, glass and ceramics industries	4	6	10	12	12	56	5	9	14	15	14	43
Workers in ferrous and metallurgical industries	7	9	15	16	14	40	8	14	20	18	14	26
Chemical workers	6	8	11	13	14	48	6	11	17	17	15	35

	Marriage 1920–4 number of children						Marriage 1925–9 number of children					
	0	1	2	3	4	5+	0	1	2	3	4	5+
Textile workers	6	9	14	14	14	43	7	13	18	17	14	31
Workers in paper industry	7	8	13	12	13	47	7	12	17	16	14	34
Workers in printing industry	11	14	21	18	13	24	13	22	26	16	9	13
Workers in tanning and leather goods industries	9	9	14	15	13	39	9	14	19	17	13	27
Workers in woodworking, carving and toy industries	6	9	14	15	14	42	7	14	20	17	14	29
Workers in food industry	8	8	12	14	13	44	9	12	18	17	13	30
Workers in clothing industry	8	10	15	15	14	38	10	16	22	17	12	23
Construction workers	6	6	11	12	12	53	6	9	14	15	14	42
Other blue-collar (incl. domestic helps)	7	9	13	14	13	44	8	12	18	17	14	32
All co-habiting married couples	7	9	13	14	12	45	9	14	19	16	13	29

Occupational group	Marriage 1920–4 number of children						Marriage 1925–9 number of children					
	0	1	2	3	4	5+	0	1	2	3	4	5+
Agriculture												
Self-employed peasants, gardeners, fishermen, etc.	9	14	22	19	13	22	10	16	26	20	13	16
Blue-collar workers in agriculture, etc.	8	13	19	17	14	29	10	16	22	18	13	21
Self-employed												
Self-employed artisans and craftsmen	16	23	26	16	9	9	19	25	28	15	7	6
Self-employed in other industrial occupations and crafts	20	26	27	15	7	5	23	27	27	13	6	4
Self-employed in trade	23	28	25	13	5	5	27	29	25	11	4	3
Self-employed in transport	19	26	25	14	7	9	20	27	26	15	7	5

continued on p. 212

Table 17: *continued*

	0	1	2	3	4	5+	0	1	2	3	4	5+
Self-employed in hotels and catering	22	26	26	14	7	6	28	27	25	12	5	3
Self-employed doctors	19	19	28	19	10	6	21	19	27	19	9	5
Self-employed apothecaries	25	26	28	14	4	2	26	22	27	17	5	2
Self-employed writers, freelance scholars, etc.	38	23	24	8	3	4	41	26	19	9	3	2
Self-employed artists, actors, etc.	35	28	19	9	4	4	41	27	19	8	3	2
Self-employed lawyers and notaries	23	22	28	18	6	4	23	21	29	17	7	3
Public officials and all holding official status												
Army and navy officers, etc.	20	27	30	15	6	2	24	24	29	15	6	2
Army NCOs, etc.	18	28	25	14	9	6	21	28	25	14	7	5
Church officials	13	14	22	19	15	17	13	11	20	24	16	15
Train drivers, guards, etc.	14	27	27	15	8	8	23	31	25	12	5	4
Other officials of Imperial Post Office and Railways	18	30	26	14	6	6	24	30	25	12	5	4
Doctors	19	19	27	19	10	6	22	18	24	20	10	6
University rectors and lecturers	22	18	29	17	8	5	24	18	23	19	10	5
Senior secondary school teachers and headmasters	19	25	30	16	6	3	23	22	29	16	7	3
Primary school teachers, etc.	14	27	31	16	7	5	16	25	32	17	7	4
Judges, lawyers, junior barristers	24	24	28	16	6	3	25	22	27	15	8	3
Police officers, etc.	20	30	26	15	5	4	24	27	28	14	5	3
Policemen	19	31	27	13	5	4	23	32	27	11	4	2
Other officials (mainly in admin. and bureaucracy)	21	31	27	13	5	4	24	29	27	13	5	3

	23	15	27	17	10	9	20	21	26	15	12	7
White-collar workers												
Salaried doctors	23	35	25	10	4	3	27	34	25	9	3	2
Book-keepers, others in financial administration, etc.	22	33	27	11	4	3	25	31	27	11	4	2
White-collar foremen	18	31	26	13	6	6	23	33	25	11	5	3
Other white-collar (mainly admin. and bureaucracy)	22	32	25	11	5	4	27	32	24	10	4	3
Blue-collar workers												
Miners and others in mining industry	8	18	25	19	12	18	10	23	28	18	10	11
Workers in stone, glass and ceramics industries	9	19	24	18	12	18	11	23	26	17	10	12
Workers in ferrous and metallurgical industries	15	28	26	14	8	9	18	32	26	13	6	6
Chemical workers	12	24	25	16	10	13	15	27	26	15	8	9
Textile workers	15	28	25	14	8	10	18	32	25	12	6	7
Workers in paper industry	13	23	25	16	10	13	15	27	27	15	8	8
Workers in printing industry	24	35	23	10	4	3	28	36	22	8	3	2
Workers in tanning and leather goods industries	15	27	26	15	8	9	17	30	26	14	6	6
Workers in woodworkings carving and toy industries	14	24	25	16	9	11	16	27	27	15	8	8
Workers in food industry	17	24	24	15	9	11	18	28	26	14	7	7
Workers in clothing industry	19	28	23	14	7	9	21	30	24	12	6	6
Construction workers	12	18	22	17	11	20	13	22	24	16	10	14
Other blue-collar (incl. domestic helps)	16	25	24	15	9	12	19	27	24	14	8	9
All co-habiting married couples	17	24	24	15	9	12	19	26	25	14	8	8

Source: As Table 14.

Appendix

Table 18: Regional distribution of doctors and members of statutory sickness insurance funds in the German Reich in 1885–7 and 1907–9

Region (Prussian provinces and selected German states)	Doctors 1887	Members of sickness insurance funds (1000s) 1885	Doctors 1909	Members of sickness insurance funds (1000s) 1907
East Prussia	396	50	687	171
West Prussia	301	48	518	150
Berlin	1104	252	1881	805
Brandenburg (excl. Berlin)	658	206	2571	645
Pommerania	399	73	644	206
Posen	352	46	627	157
Silesia	1108	322	1828	758
Saxony	777	264	1323	700
Schleswig-Holstein	431	110	787	363
Hanover	812	135	1316	470
Westphalia	677	191	1429	571
Hesse-Nassau	735	118	1575	427
Rhineland	1509	442	3087	1332
Hohenzollern	25	5	26	11
Kingdom of Prussia	**9284**	**2263**	**18299**	**6765**
Kingdom of Bavaria	1916	371	3451	1060
Kingdom of Saxony	1110	556	2287	1435
Württemberg	576	152	1050	413
Baden	618	131	1157	522
Hesse	388	102	720	285
Mecklenburg-Schwerin	193	26	292	78
Saxony-Weimar	120	21	230	94
Oldenburg	114	15	162	55
Brunswick	149	51	264	161
Bremen	84	18	194	76
Hamburg	302	257	770	356

Sources: Statistisches Jahrbuch für das Deutsche Reich, vol. 8 (1887), p. 160; vol. 10 (1889), p. 154; vol. 30 (1909), pp. 330–1; vol. 35 (1914), p. 441.

Appendix

Table 19: Distribution of 'quacks' in Prussian administrative districts and their ratio to doctors in 1903 and 1913

Administrative district	Number of 'quacks'		Number of 'quacks' for every 100 doctors	
	1903	1913	1903	1913
Königsberg	104	81	81	17
Gumbinnen	113	68	56	45
Danzig	145	21	46	7
Marienwerder	14	17	5	7
Berlin	1013	1035	35	28
Potsdam	294	132	17	12
Frankfurt/Oder	302	244	76	61
Stettin	25	31	6	8
Köslin	117	37	73	25
Stralsund	63	22	43	17
Posen	175	102	45	24
Bromberg	51	46	23	22
Breslau	192	261	19	24
Liegnitz	212	319	45	69
Oppeln	172	145	32	27
Magdeburg	300	308	49	52
Merseburg	142	199	25	34
Erfurt	62	85	28	38
Schleswig	307	158	36	18
Hanover	93	200	20	45
Hildesheim	66	30	21	10
Lüneburg	100	91	50	44
Stade	40	19	29	14
Osnabrück	22	10	15	8
Aurich	36	24	16	10
Münster	48	64	15	17
Minden	62	99	22	32
Arnsberg	36	224	4	26
Kassel	105	57	22	11
Wiesbaden	106	423	11	39
Cologne	86	163	10	17
Düsseldorf	310	599	25	38
Koblenz	78	59	21	16
Aachen	60	100	22	35
Trier	96	112	31	34
Sigmaringen	1	–	3	–
Prussia	5148	5610	28	28

Sources: *Das Gesundheitswesen des Preußischen Staates im Jahre 1903*, compiled by Die Medizinal-Abteilung des Ministeriums der geistlichen, Unterrichts- und Medizinal-Angelegenheiten (Berlin, 1905), p. 437. *Das Gesundheitswesen des Preußischen Staates im Jahre 1913* (Berlin, 1915), pp. 467–8.

Appendix

Table 20: Members of statutory sickness insurance funds in the German Reich 1885–1911

	Number of sickness insurance funds	Members of funds 1000s	% of popn.	% of population in funds in		
				Berlin	Province of Posen	Kingdom of Saxony
1885	18,942	4,294.2	9.2	19.2	2.7	17.5
1890	20,568	6,579.5	13.3	23.5	4.4	25.4
1895	21,362	7,525.5	14.4	24.2	4.9	25.4
1900	22,508	9,520.8	16.9	29.0	5.9	27.9
1905	22,695	11,184.5	18.4	36.1	7.2	29.5
1910	22,843	13,069.4	20.2	41.6	7.8	32.8
1911	22,778	13,619.0	20.8	43.4	8.1	33.9

If members of the sickness insurance funds for miners, which Reich insurance legislation did not include, are added to the total for members of all funds, the figures are as follows:

	Members of sickness insurance funds	
	1000s	% of population
1885	4,671.0	10.0
1890	7,018.5	14.2
1895	8,005.8	15.3
1900	10,159.2	18.0
1905	11,903.9	19.6

Source: 'Jährliche Nachweisungen über die Krankenversicherung', *Statistik des Deutschen Reichs* (new series), vols. 24, 59, 90, 140, 177, 248, 258. For data on miners, see ibid., vol. 177, pp. 38–9.

Appendix

Table 21: Number of hospital patients and mortality in Prussian administrative districts in 1880 and 1913

Administrative district (1)	Number of hospital patients[1] per 10,000 inhabitants		% increase 1880–1913 (4)	Number of deaths[2] per 10,000 inhabitants		% decrease 1880–1913 (7)
	1880 (2)	1913 (3)		1880 (5)	1913 (6)	
Königsberg	77	367	377	269	177	34
Gumbinnen	41	146	256	277	182	34
Allenstein	–	146	–	–	169	–
Danzig	138	302	119	310	184	41
Marienwerder	66	144	118	278	169	39
Berlin (city)	386	641	66	292	140	52
Potsdam	62	331	434	262	147	44
Frankfurt/Oder	45	197	338	228	162	29
Stettin	91	248	173	238	166	30
Köslin	37	148	300	213	154	28
Stralsund	139	468	237	239	177	26
Posen	59	180	205	252	162	36
Bromberg	32	156	388	261	166	36
Breslau	176	470	167	289	191	34
Liegnitz	61	267	338	282	176	38
Oppeln	158	208	32	272	191	30
Magdeburg	92	313	240	261	152	42
Merseburg	65	259	298	256	149	42
Erfurt	60	256	327	236	143	39
Schleswig	97	313	223	210	126	40
Hanover	138	372	170	231	125	46
Hildesheim	52	457	779	227	137	40
Lüneburg	70	219	213	215	128	40
Stade	35	165	371	214	131	39
Osnabrück	134	383	186	218	138	44
Aurich	22	272	1136	184	123	33
Münster	153	562	267	254	157	38
Minden	68	343	404	236	125	47
Arnsberg	86	557	548	257	137	47
Kassel	100	277	177	229	128	44
Wiesbaden	77	496	544	213	126	41
Koblenz	70	373	433	257	145	41
Düsseldorf	132	529	301	252	125	50
Cologne	168	701	317	271	145	46
Trier	79	373	372	225	138	39
Aachen	88	374	325	259	154	41
Sigmaringen	55	152	176	291	165	43
Prussia	104	368	254	254	149	41

1. Patients treated in general hospitals. Since figures are compared with average mortality rates, specialist clinics can be safely disregarded.
2. Total number of deaths (not only those in hospitals), excluding still-births.

Sources: Column 2 = *Preußische Statistik*, vol. 90 (Berlin, 1889), p. xi; Columns 3

Appendix

Table 22: Central water supply systems in German towns of at least 2,000 inhabitants *circa* 1895: comparison by size
GR = German Reich P = Prussia

Size of population	Number of towns				Number with central water supply system			
	Absolute figures		% of all towns		Absolute figures		% of all towns	
	GR	P	GR	P	GR	P	GR	P
over 10,000	341	220	21	22	296	178	87	81
5,000–10,000	372	222	23	23	231	109	62	49
3,000–5,000	479	279	29	29	217	79	45	28
2,000–3,000	435	251	27	26	133	39	31	16
Total number of towns	1,627	972			877	405		

Source: E. Grahn, *Die städtische Wasserversorgung im Deutschen Reiche, sowie in einigen Nachbarländern* (Munich and Berlin, 1902), vol. 2, no. 2, *Die Deutschen Staaten außer Preußen und Bayern*, p. viii.

---

and 6 = *Das Gesundheitswesen des Preußischen Staates im Jahre 1913*, compiled by Die Medizinal-Abteilung des Preußischen Innenministeriums (Berlin, 1915), Appendix, pp. 2 and 46; Column 5 = *Preußische Statistik*, vol. 91 (Berlin, 1887), p. v.

Appendix

Table 23: Percentage of population of Prussian administrative districts resident in places with central water supply systems in 1900

Königsberg	20
Gumbinnen	9
Danzig	32
Marienwerder	5
Berlin	97
Potsdam	42
Frankfurt/Oder	18
Stettin	26
Köslin	12
Stralsund	29
Posen	11
Bromberg	7
Breslau	38
Liegnitz	30
Oppeln	21
Magdeburg	31
Merseberg	34
Erfurt	44
Schleswig	29
Hanover	48
Hildesheim	34
Lüneberg	15
Stade	18
Osnabrück	16
Aurich	24
Münster	11
Minden	26
Arnsberg	83
Kassel	36
Wiesbaden	52
Cologne	60
Düsseldorf	70
Koblenz	52
Aachen	39
Trier	38
Sigmaringen	22
Prussia	39

Source: Das Sanitätswesen des Preußischen Staates während der Jahre 1898, 1899 und 1900, compiled by Die Medizinal-Abteilung des Ministeriums der geistlichen, Unterrichts- und Medizinal-Angelegenheiten (Berlin, 1903), pp. 386–7.

Table 24: Increase in number of towns in the German Reich with central water supply systems. Towns (at least 2,000 inhabitants) divided by size

Number of inhabitants	Absolute (and %) growth in number of towns with central water supply in each period					Number of towns	
	before 1870	1870–1880	1880–1890	1890–1900	increase up to 1900	Total	Towns still without supply in 1900
Prussia							
Under 25,000	10 (1)	35 (4)	85 (10)	154 (18)	284 (33)	857	(67)
Over 25,000	10 (10)	35 (37)	22 (23)	29 (30)	96 (100)	96	–
All towns	20 (2)	70 (8)	107 (11)	183 (19)	380 (40)	953	(60)
Other German states							
Under 25,000	10 (2)	59 (9)	116 (18)	227 (36)	412 (65)	633	(35)
Over 25,000	13 (24)	23 (43)	13 (24)	5 (9)	54 (100)	54	–
All towns	23 (3)	82 (12)	129 (19)	232 (34)	466 (68)	687	(32)
German Reich							
Under 25,000	20 (1)	94 (6)	201 (14)	381 (26)	696 (47)	1490	(53)
Over 25,000	23 (15)	58 (39)	35 (23)	34 (23)	150 (100)	150	–
All towns	43 (3)	152 (9)	236 (15)	415 (25)	846 (52)	1640	(48)

Source: E. Grahn, 'Die städtischen Wasserwerke' in R. Wuttke (ed.), *Die deutschen Städte* (Leipzig, 1904), vol. 1, p. 309.

Table 25: Average mortality rates in relation to wealth and hygiene conditions in urban districts of Berlin in 1875 and 1890

Urban district	Households with servants (%)		Housing with 5 persons or more per heated room (%)		Housing with water supply (%)		Housing with WC (%)		Housing with communal WC (%)		Average mortality (per 1000 of mean population)	
	1875	1890	1875	1890	1875	1890	1875	1890	1875	1890	1875	1890
Dorotheenstadt	42	40	7	2	54	91	31	79		32	20	16
Friedrichstadt	34	38	8	3	53	94	22	81		26	22	13
Berlin etc.	30	28	11	5	44	91	16	80		42	26	16
Friedr. W.-Stadt	28	26	7	2	51	94	18	85		40	25	–
Luisenstadt, city-side of canal	27	23	9	4	71	94	19	86		39	26	17
Luisenstadt, other side of canal	11	10	19	8	55	96	9	85		60	42	23
Suburb of Rosental	13	9	15	9	14	94	1	76		47	39	26
Wedding	8	6	23	13	–	86	–	69		42	44	30
City of Berlin	21	17	13	8	43	93	14	81		43	30	23

Sources: R. Böckh (ed.), *Die Bevölkerungs-, Gewerbe- und Wohnungs-Aufnahme vom 1. December 1875 in der Stadt Berlin* (Berlin, 1878), no. 1, part 1, p. 89; no. 2, part 2, pp. 28, 47, 62; idem, *Die Bevölkerungs- und Wohnungs-Aufnahme vom 1. December 1890 in der Stadt Berlin* (Berlin, 1896), pp. 26, 50, 60; *Statistisches Jahrbuch der Stadt Berlin*, vol. 16–17 (1889–90), p. 101.

Bibliography

Abholz, H.-H., 'Welche Bedeutung hat die Medizin für die Gesundheit?', in H.-U. Deppe (ed.), *Vernachlässigte Gesundheit*, Cologne, 1980
Ackerknecht, E.H., and E. Fischer-Homberger, 'Five Made It — One Not. The Rise of Medical Craftsmen to Academic Status during the 19th Century', in *Clio Medica*, vol. 12, 1977, pt 4
Ackerknecht, E.H., *Therapie von den Primitiven bis zum 20. Jahrhundert*, Stuttgart, 1970
——, *Geschichte und Geographie der wichtigsten Krankheiten*, Stuttgart, 1963
——, 'Anticontagionism between 1821 and 1867', in *Bulletin of the History of Medicine*, vol. 22, 1948
Alber, J., 'Zur historischen Entwicklung des Wohlfahrtsstaates in Westeuropa', in *Sozialwissenschaftliche Informationen für Unterricht und Studium*, vol. 12, 1983, pt 2
——, *Vom Armenhaus zum Wohlfahrtsstaat. Analysen zur Entwicklung der Sozialversicherung in Westeuropa*, Frankfurt a.M./ New York, 1982
Die Anstalten der Stadt Berlin für die öffentliche Gesundheitspflege und für den naturwissenschaftlichen Unterricht. Festschrift dargeboten den Mitgliedern der 59. Versammlung deutscher Naturforscher und Ärzte von den städtischen Behörden, Berlin, 1886
Der ärztliche Stand und die deutsche Arbeiterversicherung. Aus Anlaß der bevorstehenden Abänderung des Krankenversicherungsgesetzes zusammengestellt vom ärztlichen Lokalverein Augsburg, Augsburg, 1901
Aschenborn, 'Ärzte', in Rapmund, O. (ed.), *Das Preußische Medizinal- und Gesundheitswesen in den Jahren 1883–1908. Festschrift zur Feier des 25jährigen Bestehens des Preußischen Medizinalbeamten-Vereins*, Berlin, 1908
Baron, R., 'Weder Zuckerbrot noch Peitsche. Historische Konstitutionsbedingungen des Sozialstaats in Deutschland', in *Gesellschaft. Beiträge zur Marxschen Theorie*, vol. 12, Frankfurt a.M., 1979 (Edition Suhrkamp, vol. 865)
Baum, M., 'Grundriß der Säuglingsfürsorge', in S. Engel, *Grundriß der Säuglingskunde*, 10th edn, Munich, 1920
——, 'Ein Beitrag zur Frage der Beziehungen zwischen Kinderzahl und Kindersterblichkeit', in *Medizinische Reform*, vol. 18, 1910
Beck, U., 'Jenseits von Stand und Klasse? Soziale Ungleichheiten, gesellschaftliche Individualisierungsprozesse und die Entstehung neuer sozialer Formationen und Identitäten', in R. Kreckel (ed.), *Soziale Ungleichheiten*, Göttingen 1983 (*Soziale Welt*, Sonderband 2)
Bergmann, J., et al., 'Herrschaft, Klassenverhältnis und Schichtung', in

Bibliography

T.W. Adorno (ed.), *Spätkapitalismus oder Industriegesellschaft? Verhandlungen des deutschen Soziologentages 1968*, Stuttgart, 1969

Bericht des Großherzoglichen Obermedizinalraths an Großherzogliches Ministerium des Innern über den Zustand des Medizinalwesens im Großherzogthum Baden im Jahre 1869, Karlsruhe, 1871

Birch, H.G., and J.D. Gussow, *Disadvantaged Children: Health, Nutrition and School Failure*, New York/London, 1970

Blasius, D., 'Geschichte und Krankheit. Sozialgeschichtliche Perspektiven der Medizingeschichte', in *Geschichte und Gesellschaft*, vol. 2, 1976, pt 3

Bleker, J., 'Die Stadt als Krankheitsfaktor. Eine Analyse ärztlicher Auffassungen im 19. Jahrhundert', in *Medizinhistorisches Journal*, vol. 18, 1983, pts 1/2

Bluhm, A., 'Die Stillungsnot, ihre Ursachen und die Vorschläge zu ihrer Bekämpfung. Eine kritische Übersicht', in *Zeitschrift für soziale Medizin*, vol. 3, 1908

Böckh, R. (ed.), *Die Bevölkerungs- und Wohnungsaufnahme vom 1. December 1890 in der Stadt Berlin*, pt 1, section IV, Berlin, 1893

—— (ed.), *Die Bevölkerungs- und Wohnungs-Aufnahme vom 1. December 1885 in der Stadt Berlin*, pt 2, section IV, Berlin, 1891

——, 'Tabellen betreffend den Einfluß der Ernährungsweise auf die Kindersterblichkeit', in *Bulletin de l'Institut International de Statistique*, vol. 2, 2nd edn, 1887

—— (ed.), *Die Bevölkerungs-, Gewerbe und Wohnungs-Aufnahme vom 1. December 1875 in der Stadt Berlin*, pt 1, section I, Berlin, 1878

Böhmert, W., '100 Jahre Geburtenstatistik in Bremen nebst Angaben über die Säuglingssterblichkeit', in *Mitteilungen des Statistischen Landesamts Bremen im Jahre 1926*, Bremen, 1926, pt 3

Bollinger, O. von, *Wandlungen der Medizin und des Ärztestandes in den letzten 50 Jahren*, Munich, 1909

Bolte, K.M., et al., *Bevölkerung. Statistik, Theorie, Geschichte und Politik des Bevölkerungsprozesses*, 4th edn, Opladen, 1980 (utb, vol. 986)

Borchardt, K., 'Regionale Wachstumsdifferenzierung in Deutschland im 19. Jahrhundert unter besonderer Berücksichtigung des West-Ost-Gefälles', in W. Abel et al. (eds), *Wirtschaft, Geschichte und Wirtschaftsgeschichte. Festschrift zum 65. Geburtstag von Friedrich Lütge*, Stuttgart, 1966

Borscheid, P., and H. Schomerus, 'Mobilität und soziale Lage der württembergischen Fabrikarbeiterschaft im 19. Jahrhundert', in P.J. Müller (ed.), *Die Analyse prozeß-produzierter Daten*, Stuttgart, 1977

Branca, P. (ed.), *The Medicine Show: Patients, Physicians and the Perplexities of the Health Revolution in Modern Society*, New York, 1977

Branca, P., *Silent Sisterhood: Middle-Class Women in the Victorian Home*, London, 1975

Bronfenbrenner, U., 'Ökologische Sozialisationsforschung — Ein Bezugsrahmen', in idem, *Ökologische Sozialisationsforschung*, Stuttgart, 1976

Brügelmann, J., 'Medikalisierung von Säuglings- und Erwachsenenalter in Deutschland zu Beginn des 19. Jahrhunderts aufgrund von medizinischen Topographien', in A.E. Imhof (ed.), *Leib und Leben in der Geschichte der Neuzeit*, Berlin, 1983

——, 'Der Blick des Arztes auf die Krankheit im Alltag 1779–1850. Medizinische Topographien als Quelle für die Sozialgeschichte des Gesundheitswesens, Phil. Diss., Freie Universität Berlin, 1982

——, 'Observations on the Process of Medicalization in Germany, 1770–1830, Based on Medical Topographies', in J.-P. Goubert (ed.), *La Médicalisation de la Societé Francaise 1770–1830*, Waterloo, Ont., 1982 (Historical Reflections, vol. 9, 1982, pts 1/2)

Bry, G., *Wages in Germany 1871–1945: A Study by the National Bureau of Economic Research*, Princeton, 1960

Conze, W., 'Sozialgeschichte 1850–1918', in W. Zorn (ed.), *Handbuch der deutschen Wirtschafts- und Sozialgeschichte*, vol. 2, Stuttgart, 1976

Corsi, P., and P. Weindling (eds), *Information Sources in the History of Science and Medicine*, London etc., 1983

Coyner, S.J., 'Class Consciousness and Consumption: The New Middle Class during the Weimar Republic', in *Journal of Social History*, vol. 10, 1977, pt 3

——, 'Class Patterns of Family Income and Expenditure during the Weimar Republic: German White-Collar Employees as Harbingers of Modern Society', Phil. Diss., Rutgers University, 1975

Dahrendorf, R., *Lebenschancen*, Frankfurt a.M., 1979

Desai, A.V., *Real Wages in Germany 1871–1913*, Oxford, 1968

Desplanques, G., 'L'inégalité sociale devant la mort', in *Economie et Statistique*, pt 162, January 1984

Das Deutsche Reich in gesundheitlicher und demographischer Beziehung. Festschrift, den Teilnehmern am 14. Internationalen Kongresse für Hygiene und Demographie Berlin 1907 gewidmet vom Kaiserlichen Gesundheitsamte und vom Kaiserlichen Statistischen Amte, Berlin, 1907

Dickler, R.A., 'Labor Market Pressure Aspects of Agricultural Growth in the Eastern Region of Prussia, 1840–1914: A Case Study of Economic-Demographic Interrelations during the Demographic Transition', PhD Diss., University of Pennsylvania, 1975

Duden, B., 'Keine Nachsicht gegen das schöne Geschlecht. Wie sich Ärzte die Kontrolle über Gebärmütter aneigneten', in S. von Paczensky (ed.), *Wir sind keine Mörderinnen*, Reinbek, 1980

—— and U. Ottmüller, 'Der süße Bronnen. Zur Geschichte des Stillens', in *Courage*, vol. 3, 1978, pt 2

Ende, A., 'Zur Geschichte der Stillfeindlichkeit in Deutschland (1870–1975)', in *Kindheit*, vol. 1, 1979, pt 2

Esche, P. vor dem, 'Die Versorgung der Bevölkerung mit Krankenhäusern in Deutschland von 1876 bis zur Gegenwart', in *Archiv für Hygiene*, vol. 138, 1954

——, 'Die Verbreitung der Ärzte im Deutschen Reich bzw. in der Bundesrrepublik von 1876–1950', in *Archiv für Hygiene*, vol. 138, 1954

Eulenberg, H. (ed.), *Handbuch des öffentlichen Gesundheitswesens*, vol. 1, Berlin, 1881

Evans, R.J., 'Social Inequality in the Face of Death and Disease in 19th-Century Hamburg', paper presented to the 8th UEA Research Seminar in Modern German Social History, 'Health and Medicine', Norwich: University of East Anglia, 9–10 Jan. 1985 (duplicated MS)

——, 'Die Cholera und die Sozialdemokratie: Arbeiterbewegung, Bürgertum und Staat in Hamburg während der Krise von 1892', in A. Herzig et al. (eds), *Arbeiter in Hamburg*, Hamburg, 1983

Ferber, C. von, *Soziologie für Mediziner. Eine Einführung*, Berlin etc., 1975

——, 'Volks- und Laienmedizin als Alternative zur wissenschaftlichen Medizin — Zur Partizipation im Gesundheitswesen', in *Soziale Sicherheit*, vol. 24, 1975

——, 'Gesellschaftliche Grundlagen der Volksgesundheit', in *Arbeit und Leistung*, vol. 25, 1971

Finzen, A., *Arzt, Patient und Gesellschaft. Die Orientierung der ärztlichen Berufsrolle an der sozialen Wirklichkeit*, Stuttgart, 1969 (*Medizin in Geschichte und Kultur*, vol. 10)

Fischer, A., *Geschichte des deutschen Gesundheitswesens*, 2 vols., Hildesheim, 1968 (repr. of 1st edn, 1933)

——, 'Vermißte Folgen der deutschen Sozialversicherung. Ein Beitrag zu der Frage: Schreitet die physische Verelendung der deutschen Arbeiterbevölkerung fort?', in *Jahrbücher für Nationalökonomie und Statistik*, 3rd series, vol. 46, 1913

Flatten, H., 'Die Bekämpfung der einzelnen übertragbaren Krankheiten', in R. Abel (ed.), *Handbuch der praktischen Hygiene*, vol. 1, Jena, 1913

Flinn, M.W., *The European Demographic System 1500–1820*, Brighton, 1981

Freidson, E., *Profession of Medicine. A Study of the Sociology of Applied Knowledge*, New York, 1970

Freudenberg, K., 'Fruchbarkeit und Sterblichkeit in den Berliner Verwaltungsbezirken in Beziehung zu deren sozialer Struktur', in A. Grotjahn et al. (eds), *Ergebnisse der sozialen Hygiene und Gesundheitsfürsorge*, vol. 1, Leipzig, 1929

Frevert, U., 'Professional Medicine and the Working Classes in Imperial Germany', in *Journal of Contemporary History*, vol. 20, 1985, pt 4

——, '"Fürsorgliche Belagerung": Hygienebewegung und Arbeiterfrauen im 19. und frühen 20. Jahrhundert', in *Geschichte und Gesellschaft*, vol. 11, 1985, pt 4

——, *Krankheit als politisches Problem 1770–1880. Soziale Unterschichten in Preußen zwischen medizinischer Polizei und staatlicher Sozialversicherung*, Göttingen, 1984

——, 'Frauen und Ärzte im späten 18. und frühen 19. Jahrhundert — zur Sozialgeschichte eines Gewaltverhältnisses', in A. Kuhn and J. Rüsen

(eds), *Frauen in der Geschichte II*, Düsseldorf, 1982
——, 'Arbeiterkrankheit und Arbeiterkrankenkassen im Industrialisierungsprozeß Preußens (1840–1870)', in W. Conze and U. Engelhardt (eds), *Arbeiterexistenz im 19. Jahrhundert*, Stuttgart, 1981
Funk, J., 'Die Sterblichkeit nach sozialen Klassen in der Stadt Bremen', in *Mitteilungen des Bremischen Statistischen Amts im Jahre 1911*, pt 1, Bremen, 1911
Gajewski, W., 'Statistik der Krankheiten und Gebrechen einschließlich der Krankenanstaltsstatistik', in F. Burgdörfer (ed.), *Die Statistik in Deutschland nach ihrem heutigen Stand. Ehrengabe für Friedrich Zahn*, vol. 1, Berlin, 1940
Gärtner, A., *Leitfaden der Hygiene*, 5th edn, Jena, 1909
Gebhard, H., 'Die Erfolge der Heilstätten für Lungenkranke', in B. Fränkel (ed.), *Der Stand der Tuberkulose-Bekämpfung in Deutschland*, Berlin, 1905
Gerlach, E., and K. Hünerberg, *Die Wasserversorgung*, 6th edn., enlarged, Munich/Vienna, 1963
Die Gesundheitsverhältnisse Hamburgs im 19. Jahrhundert. Den ärztlichen Teilnehmern der 73. Versammlung deutscher Naturforscher und Ärzte gewidmet von dem Medicinal-Collegium, Hamburg, 1901
Das Gesundheitswesen des Preußischen Staates im Jahre 1913, Berlin, 1915
Das Gesundheitswesen des Preußischen Staates im Jahre 1911, Berlin, 1912
Das Gesundheitswesen des Preußischen Staates im Jahre 1903, Berlin, 1905
Giddens, A., *The Class Structure of the Advanced Societies*, London, 1973
Gleichmann, P.R., 'Die Verhäuslichung körperlicher Verrichtungen', in idem et al. (eds), *Materialien zu Norbert Elias' Zivilisationstheorie*, Frankfurt a.M., 1977
Göckenjan, G., 'Medizin und Ärzte als Faktor der Disziplinierung der Unterschichten: Der Kassenarzt', in C. Sachße and F. Tennstedt (eds), *Soziale Sicherheit und soziale Disziplinierung. Beiträge zu einer historischen Theorie der Sozialpolitik*, Frankfurt a.M., 1986
——, *Kurieren und Staat machen. Gesundheit und Medizin in der bürgerlichen Welt*, Frankfurt a.M., 1985
Goerke, H., 'Personelle und arbeitstechnische Gegebenheiten im Krankenhaus des 19. Jahrhunderts', in *Studien zur Krankenhausgeschichte im 19. Jahrhundert im Hinblick auf die Entwicklung in Deutschland*, Göttingen, 1976
Gottstein, A., *Das Heilwesen der Gegenwart*, Berlin, 1924
——, *Geschichte der Hygiene im neunzehnten Jahrhundert*, Berlin, 1901
Goubert, J.-P., 'Public Hygiene and Mortality Decline in France in the 19th Century', in T. Bengtsson et al. (eds), *Pre-Industrial Population Change. The Mortality Decline and Short-Term Population Movements*, Stockholm, 1984
Gransche, E., and E. Rothenbacher, *Langfristige Entwicklungstendenzen der Wohnverhältnisse in Deutschland 1861–1910*, Universität Mannheim, 1985

Bibliography

(SFB 3, Arbeitspapier 158, duplicated MS)
Greer, A.L., and S. Greer (eds), *Cities and Sickness. Health Care in Urban America*, Beverly Hills etc., 1983
Grotjahn, A., *Soziale Pathologie*, 3rd edn., Berlin, 1923
—— and J. Kaup (eds), *Handwörterbuch der Sozialen Hygiene*, vol. 1, Leipzig, 1912
Günther, A., *Lebenshaltung des Mittelstandes. Statistische und theoretische Untersuchungen zur Konsumtionslehre*, Munich/Leipzig, 1920 (*Schriften des Vereins für Sozialpolitik*, vol. 146)
——, 'Die deutschen Techniker', in *Soziale Praxis und Archiv für Volkswohlfahrt*, vol. 21, 1911/12, pt 20
Haines, M., *Fertility and Occupation. Population Patterns in Industrialization*, New York etc., 1979
Haller, M., *Theorie der Klassenbildung und sozialen Schichtung*, Frankfurt a.M./New York, 1983
——, *Klassenbildung und soziale Schichtung in Österreich. Analysen zur Sozialstruktur, sozialen Ungleichheit und Mobilität*, Frankfurt a.M./New York, 1982
Hamburger, C., 'Beitrag zu der Frage, ob Kinderzahl und Kindersterblichkeit zusammenhängen', in *Klinische Wochenschrift*, vol. 53, 1916, pt 47, 2nd half-year
——, 'Uber den Zusammenhang zwischen Konzeptionsziffer und Kindersterblichkeit in (großstädtischen) Arbeiterkreisen', in *Zeitschrift für soziale Medizin*, vol. 3, 1908
Handl, J., et al., *Klassenlagen und Sozialstruktur. Empirische Untersuchungen für die Bundesrepublik Deutschland*, Frankfurt a.M., 1977
Hansen, E., et al., *Seit über einem Jahrhundert . . . : Verschüttete Alternativen in der Sozialpolitik*, Cologne, 1981
Hartmann, F., *Wandel und Bestand in der Heilkunde T. I.* (Materialien zur Geschichte der Medizin für Studenten), Munich etc., 1977
Helberger, C., 'Soziale Indikatoren für das Gesundheitswesen der BRD. Ansätze, Probleme, Ergebnisse', in *Allgemeines Statistisches Archiv*, vol. 60, 1976, pt 1
Herrlitz, H.-G., and H. Titze, 'Überfüllung als bildungspolitische Strategie. Zur administrativen Steuerung der Lehrerarbeitslosigkeit in Preußen 1870–1914', in *Die Deutsche Schule*, vol. 68, 1976
Historia Hospitalium. Zeitschrift der Deutschen Gesellschaft für Krankenhausgeschichte, pt 13, 1979/80
Hoffmann, W.G., et al., *Das Wachstum der deutschen Wirtschaft seit der Mitte des 19. Jahrhunderts*, Berlin etc., 1965
Höhn, C., et. al. (eds), *Determinants of Fertility Trends: Theories Reexamined*, Lüttich, 1982
Hohorst, G., 'The Decline of Fertility Once Again: A Critical Note, on John Knodel's Book and Standardized Demographic Indexes, in *Historical Social Research — Quantum Information*, pt 22, 1982

Bibliography

Hopkins, D.R., *Princes and Peasants. Smallpox in History*, Chicago/London, 1983

Huerkamp, C., 'The History of Smallpox Vaccination in Germany: A First Step in the Medicalization of the General Public', in *Journal of Contemporary History*, vol. 20, 1985, pt 4

——, *Der Aufstieg der Ärzte im 19. Jahrhundert. Vom gelehrten Stand zum professionellen Experten: Das Beispiel Preußens*, Göttingen, 1985

——, 'Die preußisch-deutsche Ärzteschaft als Teil des Bildungsbürgertums: Wandel in Lage und Selbstverständnis vom ausgehenden 18. Jahrhundert bis zum Kaiserreich', in W. Conze and J. Kocka (eds), *Bildungsbürgertum im 19. Jahrhundert, Teil 1: Bildungsbürgertum und Professionalisierung in internationalen Vergleichen*, Stuttgart, 1985.

—— and R. Spree, 'Arbeitsmarktstrategien der deutschen Ärtzteschaft im späten 19. und frühen 20. Jahrhundert. Zur Entwicklung des Marktes für professionelle ärztliche Dienstleistungen', in T. Pierenkemper and R.H. Tilly (eds), *Historische Arbeitsmarktforschung*, Göttingen, 1982

——, 'Ärzte und Professionalisierung in Deutschland. Überlegungen zum Wandel des Arztberufs im 19. Jahrhundert', in *Geschichte und Gesellschaft*, vol. 6, 1980, pt 3

Illich, I., *Medical Nemesis*, London, 1975

Imhof, A.E., *Die gewonnenen Jahre. Von der Zunahme unserer Lebensspanne seit dreihundert Jahren*, Munich, 1981

——, 'Unterschiedliche Säuglingssterblichkeit in Deutschland' 18. bis 20. Jahrhundert — Warum?', in *Zeitschrift für Bevölkerungswisenschaft*, vol. 7, 1981, pt 3

—— (ed.), *Mensch und Gesundheit in der Geschichte. Vorträge eines internationalen Colloquiums in Berlin vom 20. bis zum 23. September 1978*, Husum, 1980 (*Abhandlungen zur Geschichte der Medizin und der Naturwissenschaften*, pt 39)

—— (ed.), *Biologie des Menschen in der Geschichte. Beiträge zur Sozialgeschichte der Neuzeit aus Frankreich und Skandinavien*, Stuttgart–Bad Cannstatt, 1978 (*Kultur und Gesellschaft*, vol. 3)

——, *Einführung in die Historische Demographie*, Munich, 1977

——, 'The Hospital in the 18th Century: For Whom?', in *Journal of Social History*, vol. 10, 1977, pt 4

—— and O. Larsen, *Sozialgeschichte und Medizin. Probleme der quantifizierenden Quellenbearbeitung in der Sozial- und Medizingeschichte*, Oslo/Stuttgart, 1976

——, *Historische Demographie als Sozialgeschichte*, 2 vols., Darmstadt/Marburg, 1975

Jaenicke, C., 'Landesversicherungsanstalten und Tuberkulosebekämpfung, mit besonderer Berücksichtigung der Tätigkeit der Landesversicherungsanstalt Thüringen', in K.H. Blümel (ed.), *Handbuch der Tuberkulose-Fürsorge*, vol. 1, Munich, 1926

Jeck, A., *Wachstum und Verteilung des Volkseinkommens*, Tübingen, 1970

Jetter, D., *Grundzüge der Krankenhausgeschichte (1800–1900)*, Darmstadt, 1977

Kadritzke, U., *Angestellte — Die geduldigen Arbeiter. Zur Soziologie und sozialen Bewegung der Angestellten*, Frankfurt/Cologne, 1975

Kaelble, H., *Industrialisation and Social Inequality in 19th-Century Europe*, Leamington Spa, 1985

Kaiserliches Gesundheitsamt (eds), *Blattern und Schutzpockenimfung. Denkschrift zur Beurteilung des Nutzens des Impfgesetzes und zur Würdigung der dagegen gerichteten Angriffe*, Berlin, 1896

Kater, M.H., 'Professionalization and Socialization of Physicians in Wilhelmine and Weimar Germany', in *Journal of Contemporary History*, vol. 20, 1985, pt 4

Kaupen-Haas, H., 'Gesundheitsverhalten und Krankheitsverhalten aus historischer Sicht. Zwei Strategien zur Gesundheitssicherung', in *Jahrbuch für kritische Medizin*, vol. 1, Berlin, 1976

Kayserling, A., 'Die Tuberkulose-Assanierung Berlins', in *Archiv für Soziale Hygiene*, vol. 6, 1911

——, 'Die Tuberkulose in ihrem Verhältnis zur Mortalität in Deutschland', in B. Fränkel (ed.), Der Stand der Tuberkulose-Bekämpfung in Deutschland, Berlin, 1905

Kintner, H.J., 'The Determinants of Infant Mortality in Germany from 1871 to 1933', PhD Diss., University of Michigan, 1982 (xerox)

Kirchner, —, 'Die Seuchenbekämpfung unter Berücksichtigung der einschlägigen deutschen und preußischen Gesetzgebung', in O. Rapmund (ed.), *Das Preußische Medizinal- und Gesundheitswesen in den Jahren 1883–1908*, Berlin, 1908

Knodel, J., 'Demographic Transitions in German Villages', in A.J. Coale and S. Watkins (eds), *The Decline of European Fertility*, Princeton, NJ (forthcoming)

——, *Seasonal Variation in Infant Mortality: An Approach with Applications*, University of Michigan, Population Studies Center, 1982 (Research Report, nos. 28–9).

——, 'Child Mortality and Reproductive Behaviour in German Village Populations in the Past: A Micro-Level Analysis of the Replacement Effect', in *Population Studies*, vol. 36, 1982, pt 2

—— and C. Wilson, 'The Secular Increase in Fecundity in German Village Populations: An Analysis of Reproductive Histories of Couples Married 1750–1899', in *Population Studies*, vol. 35, 1981, pt 1

——, 'Breast-Feeding and Population Growth', in *Science*, vol. 198, 1977

—— and H. Kintner, 'The Impact of Breast-Feeding Patterns on the Biometric Analysis of Infant Mortality', in *Demography*, vol. 14, 1977

——, *The Decline of Fertility in Germany, 1871–1939*, Princeton, NJ, 1974

——, 'Infant Mortality in Three Bavarian Villages: An Analysis of Family Histories from the 19th Century', in *Population Studies*, vol. 22, 1968

Koch, K.H., 'Die Kinderzahlen der Arbeiter und Angestellten von Kieler

Werften', in *Archiv für Rassen- und Gesellschaftsbiologie*, vol. 31, 1937

Kocka, J., *Die Angestellten in der deutschen Geschichte 1850–1980. Vom Privatbeamten zum angestellten Arbeitnehmer*, Göttingen, 1981

——, *Angestellte zwischen Faschismus und Demokratie. Zur politischen Sozialgeschichte der Angestellten: USA 1890–1940 im internationalen Vergleich*, Göttingen, 1977

——, 'Theorien in der Sozial- und Gesellschaftsgeschichte. Vorschläge zur historischen Schichtungsanalyse', in *Geschichte und Gesellschaft*, vol. 1, 1975, pt 1

——, 'Vorindustrielle Faktoren in der deutschen Industrialisierung. Industriebürokratie und "neuer Mittelstand"', in M. Stürmer (ed.), *Das kaiserliche Deutschland*, Düsseldorf, 1970

Köhler, P.A., and H.F. Zacher (eds), *Beiträge zu Geschichte und aktueller Situation der Sozialversicherung*, Berlin, 1983

——, —— (eds), *Ein Jahrhundert Sozialversicherung in der Bundesrepublik Deutschland, Frankreich, Großbritannien, Österreich und der Schweiz*, Berlin, 1981

Kohn, R., and K.L. White (eds), *Health Care. An International Study*, London etc., 1976

Komitee zur Ermittlung der Säuglingsernährung in Hannover-Linden, *Säuglingsernährung, Säuglingssterblichkeit und Säuglingsschutz in den Städten Hannover und Linden*, Berlin, n.d. [1913]

'Die Krankenversicherung im Jahre 1900', in *Statistik des Deutschen Reichs*, N.F., vol. 140, Berlin, 1903

Krankheits- und Sterblichkeitsverhältnisse in der Ortskrankenkasse für Leipzig und Umgegend. Bearbeitet im Kaiserlichen Statistischen Amte, 4 vols., Berlin, 1910

Kreckel, R. (ed.), *Soziale Ungleichheiten*, Göttingen, 1983 (*Soziale Welt*, Sonderband 2)

Kriege, ——, and — Seutemann, 'Ernährungsverhältnisse und Sterblichkeit der Säuglinge in Barmen', in *Centralblatt für allgemeine Gesundheitspflege*, vol. 25, 1906

Kruse, W., 'Die Verminderung der Sterblichkeit in den letzten Jahrzehnten und ihr jetziger Stand', in *Zeitschrift für Hygiene und Infectionskrankheiten*, vol. 25, 1897

Kübler, P., *Geschichte der Pocken und der Impfung*, Berlin, 1901

Kuczinsky, J., *Darstellung der Lage der Arbeiter in Deutschland von 1871 bis 1900*, Berlin, 1962 (*Die Geschichte der Lage der Arbeiter unter dem Kapitalismus*, vol. 3)

Kunitz, S.J., 'Speculations on the European Mortality Decline', in *Economic History Review*, 2nd series, vol. 36, 1983, pt 3

Labisch, A., '"Hygiene ist Moral — Moral ist Hygiene" — Soziale Disziplinierung durch Ärzte und Medizin', in C. Sachße and F. Tennstedt (eds), *Soziale Sicherheit und soziale Disziplinierung, Beiträge zu einer historischen Theorie der Sozialpolitik*, Frankfurt a.M., 1986

―――, 'Die soziale Konstruktion der "Gesundheit" und des "Homo Hygienicus": Zur Soziogenese eines sozialen Gutes', in *Österreichische Zeitschrift für Soziologie*, vol. 10, 1985, pts 3/4

―――, 'Doctors, Workers and the Scientific Cosmology of the Industrial World: The Social Construction of "Health" and the "Homo Hygienicus", in *Journal of Contemporary History*, vol. 20, 1985, pt 4

―――, 'Entwicklungslinien des öffentlichen Gesundheitsdienstes in Deutschland. Vorüberlegungen zur historischen Soziologie öffentlicher Gesundheitsvorsorge', in *Das öffentliche Gesundheitswesen*, vol. 44, 1982

―――, 'Das Krankenhaus in der Gesundheitspolitik der deutschen Sozialdemokratie vor dem Ersten Weltkrieg', in *Medizinsoziologisches Jahrbuch*, vol. 1, 1981

―――, 'Sozialgeschichte der Medizin. Methodologische Überlegungen und Forschungsbericht', in *Archiv für Sozialgeschichte*, vol. 20, 1980

―――, 'Ärzte und Arbeiterbewegung', in *Medizinsoziologische Mitteilungen*, vol. 3, 1977, pt 4

―――, 'Die gesundheitspolitischen Vorstellungen der deutschen Sozialdemokratie von ihrer Gründung bis zur Parteispaltung (1863–1917)', in *Archiv für Sozialgeschichte*, vol. 16, 1976

Lee, W.R., 'The Impact of Agrarian Change on Women's Work and Child Care in Early-Nineteenth-Century Prussia', in J.C. Fout (ed.), *German Women in the Nineteenth Century: A Social History*, New York/London, 1984

―――, 'Family and "Modernisation": The Peasant Family and Social Change in Nineteenth-Century Bavaria', in R. Evans and W.R. Lee (eds), *The German Family*, London, 1981

―――, 'The Mechanism of Mortality Change in Germany, 1750–1850', in *Medizinhistorisches Journal*, vol. 15, 1980, pt 3

―――, 'Germany', in idem (ed.), *European Demography and Economic Growth*, London, 1979

―――, 'Regional Differences in the Population Growth of Germany in the Early 19th Century', in R. Fremdling and R.H. Tilly (eds), *Industrialisierung und Raum. Studien zur regionalen Differenzierung im Deutschland des 19. Jahrhunderts*, Stuttgart, 1979

―――, 'Primary Sector Output and Mortality Changes in Early-19th-Century Bavaria', in *Journal of European Economic History*, vol. 6, 1977

Linde, H., 'Familie und Haushalt als Gegenstand bevölkerungsgeschichtlicher Forschung. Erörterung eines problembezogenen und materialorientierten Bezugsrahmens', in W. Conze (ed.), *Sozialgeschichte der Familie in der Neuzeit Europas. Neue Forschungen*, Stuttgart, 1976

Littrow, C. von, 'Die Stellung des Deutschen Ärztetages zur Kurpfuscherfrage in Deutschland von 1869 bis 1908', in *Wissenschaftliche Zeitschrift der Humboldt-Universität zu Berlin, Mathematisch-Naturwissenschaftliche Reihe*, vol. 19, 1970, pt 4

―――, 'Der Deutsche Ärztetag und die Kurpfuscherfrage. (Ein Beitrag zur

Geschichte der Kurpfuscherei in Deutschland von 1869 bis 1908)', Diss., Humboldt-Universität, Berlin, 1969

Luckin, B., 'Evaluating the Sanitary Revolution: Typhus and Typhoid in London, 1851–1900', in R. Woods and J. Woodward (eds), *Urban Disease and Mortality in Nineteenth-Century England*, London/New York, 1984

——, 'Death and Survival in the City: Approaches to the History of Disease', in *Urban History Yearbook*, 1980

——, 'The Final Catastrophe — Cholera in London, 1866, in *Medical History*, vol. 21, 1977, pt 1

Mackenroth, G., *Bevölkerungslehre*, Berlin, 1953

MacKeown, T., *The Role of Medicine: Dream, Mirage or Nemesis?*, London, 1979

——, *The Modern Rise of Population*, London, 1976

—— and R.G. Record, 'Reasons for the Decline of Mortality in England and Wales during the Nineteenth Century', in *Population Studies*, vol. 16, 1962

McKinlay, J.B., (ed.), 'Mortality, Morbidity, and the Inverse Care Law', in A.L. Greer and S. Greer (eds), *Cities and Sickness, Health Care in Urban America*, Beverly Hills etc., 1983

McNeill, W.H., *Seuchen machen Geschichte. Geißeln der Völker*, Munich, 1978

Marschalck, P., *Bevölkerungsgeschichte Deutschlands im 19. und 20. Jahrhundert*, Frankfurt a.M., 1984

Marx, C., *Die Entwickelung des ärztlichen Standes seit den ersten Dezennie des 19. Jahrhunderts*, Berlin, 1907

Medizinal-statistische Mitteilungen aus dem Kaiserlichen Gesundheitsamte, vol. 19, Berlin, 1917

Meerwarth, R., 'Die Entwicklung der Bevölkerung in Deutschland während der Kriegs- und Nachkriegszeit', in idem et al., *Die Einwirkung des Krieges auf Bevölkerungsbewegung, Einkommen und Lebenshaltung in Deutschland*, Stuttgart etc., 1932

Meier, E., 'Statistik der Todesursachen', in F. Burgdörfer (ed.), *Die Statistik in Deutschland nach ihrem heutigen Stand*, vol. 1, Berlin, 1940

Möllers, B., 'Deutsche Tuberkulosestatistik', in K.H. Blümel (ed.), *Handbuch der Tuberkulose-Fürsorge*, vol. 1, Munich, 1926

Mommsen, W.J., and W. Mock (eds), *The Origins of the Welfare State in Britain and Germany*, London, 1982

Müller, D.K., 'Qualifikationskrise und Schulreform', in U. Herrmann (ed.), *Historische Pädagogik*, Weinheim/Basle, 1977 (*Zeitschrift für Pädagogik*, Beiheft 14)

Müller, J., 'Geburtenrückgang', in *Handwörterbuch der Staatswissenschaften*, 4th edn., vol. 4, Jena, 1927

Müller, R., and D. Milles (eds), *Beiträge zur Geschichte der Arbeiterkrankheiten und der Arbeitsmedizin in Deutschland*, Dortmund, 1984 (*Schriften-*

reihe der Bundesanstalt für Arbeitsschutz, Sonderschrift 15)

Müller, S.F., 'Mittelständische Schulpolitik. Die Rezeption des Überfüllungsproblems im gewerblichen und Bildungsbürgertum am Ende des 19. Jahrhunderts', in U. Herrmann (ed.), *Historische Pädagogik*, Weinheim/Basle, 1977

Müller, W., et al., *Strukturwandel der Frauenarbeit 1880–1980*, Frankfurt/New York, 1983

Naschold, F., *Kassenärzte und Krankenversicherungsreform. Zu einer Theorie der Statuspolitik*, Freiburg i.Br., 1967

Nell, A. von, 'Die Entwicklung der generativen Strukturen bürgerlicher und bäuerlicher Familien von 1750 bis zur Gegenwart', Diss., Bochum, 1973

Niethammer, L. (ed.), *Wohnen im Wandel*, Wuppertal, 1979

—— and F. Brüggemeier, 'Wie wohnten Arbeiter im Kaiserreich?', in *Archiv für Sozialgeschichte*, vol. 16, 1976

Offe, C., 'Tauschverhältnis und politische Steuerung. Zur Aktualität des Legitimationsproblems', in C. Offe, *Strukturprobleme des kapitalistischen Staates*, Frankfurt a.M., 1972

Omram, A., 'Epidemiologic Transition in the U.S. The Health Factor in Population Change', in *Population Bulletin*, vol. 32, 1977, pt 2

——, 'The Epidemiologic Transition. A Theory of the Epidemiology of Population Change', in *Milbank Memorial Fund Quarterly*, vol. 49, 1971, pt 1

Orsagh, T.J., 'Löhne in Deutschland 1871–1913: Neuere Literatur und weitere Ergebnisse', in *Zeitschrift für die gesamte Staatswissenschaft*, vol. 125, 1969

Ottmüller, U., 'Speikinder — Gedeihkinder. Kommunikationstheoretische Überlegungen zu Gestalt und Funktion frühkindlicher Sozialisation im bäuerlichen Lebenszusammenhang des deutschsprachigen 19. u. frühen 20. Jahrhunderts', Phil. Diss., Freie Universität Berlin, 1983

——, '"Mutterpflichten" — Die Wandlungen ihrer inhaltlichen Ausformung durch die akademische Medizin', in *Gesellschaft, Beiträge zur Marxschen Theorie*, vol. 14, Frankfurt a.M., 1981

——, 'Mutter und Wickelkind in der vormedikalisierten Gesellschaft des deutschsprachigen Raums (ab ca. 1500)', in *Beiträge zur feministischen Theorie und Praxis*, pt 5, 1981

——, 'Mutterschaft und romantische Liebe. Alltagsweltliche Ideologien der Familie und ihre praktischen Konsequenzen', in *Sozialwissenschaftliche Informationen für Unterricht und Studium*, vol. 8, 1979, pt 1

Parry, N., and J. Parry, *The Rise of the Medical Profession. A Study of Collective Social Mobility*, London, 1976

Pelling, M., *Cholera, Fever and English Medicine 1825–1865*, Oxford, 1978

Pflanz, M., *Sozialer Wandel und Krankheit. Ergebnisse und Probleme der medizinischen Soziologie*, Stuttgart, 1962

Plaut, T., *Der Gewerkschaftskampf der deutschen Ärzte*, Karlsruhe, 1913

Bibliography

Pompey, H., '"Pastoralmedizin" — der Beitrag der Seelsorge zur psychophysischen Gesundheit', in A.E. Imhof (ed.), *Mensch und Gesundheit in der Geschichte*, Husum, 1980

Poppel, F.W.A. van, *Differential Fertility in the Netherlands: An Overview of Long-Term Trends with Special Reference to the Post-World War I Marriage Cohorts*, Netherlands Interuniversity Demographic Institute, Voorburg, 1983 (Working Paper 39)

Presse- und Informationsamt der Bundesregierung (eds), *Gesellschaftliche Daten 1979*, Bonn, 1979

Preston, S.H. (ed.), *The Effects of Infant and Child Mortality on Fertility*, New York, 1977

——, *Mortality Patterns in National Populations: With Special Reference to Recorded Causes of Death*, New York etc., 1976

Prinzing, F., *Handbuch der medizinischen Statistik*, 1st edn., Jena 1906; 2nd edn., Jena, 1931

——, 'Die Gesundheitsstatistik', in R. Abel (ed.), *Handbuch der praktischen Hygiene*, vol. 1, Jena, 1913

——, 'Die Entwicklung der Kindersterblichkeit in den europäischen Staaten', in *Jahrbücher für Nationalökonomie und Statistik*, 3rd series, vol. 17, 1899

Razzell, P.E., *The Impact of Inoculation on Smallpox Mortality in Eighteenth-Century Britain*, Brighton, 1977

——, '"An Interpretation of the Modern Rise of Population in Europe" — A Critique', in *Population Studies*, vol. 28, 1974, pt 1

Reuter, H.-G., 'Verteilungs- und Umverteilungseffekte der Sozialversicherungsgesetzgebung im Kaiserreich', in F. Blaich (ed.), *Staatliche Umverteilungspolitik in historischer Perspektive*, Berlin, 1980

Ringer, F., *Education and Society in Modern Europe*, Bloomington/London 1979

Ritter, G.A., *Social Welfare in Germany and Britain*, Leamington Spa, 1985

—— and J. Kocka (eds), *Deutsche Sozialgeschichte. Dokumente und Skizzen*, vol. 2: *1870–1914*, Munich, 1974

Roesle, E., 'Die Sterblichkeit im ersten Lebensmonat. Ein internationaler, statistischer Vergleich', in *Zeitschrift für soziale Medizin*, vol. 5, 1910

Rosen, G., Economic and Social Policy in the Development of Public Health, in idem, *From Medical Police to Social Medicine: Essays on the History of Health Care*, New York, 1974

——, 'Disease, Debility, and Death', in H.J. Dyos and M. Wolff (eds), *The Victorian City. Images and Realities*, vol. 2, London/Boston, 1973

——, *A History of Public Health*, New York, 1958

Rosenfeld, S., *Die Tuberkulosestatistik*, Genf, 1925 (League of Nations Health Organisation)

——, 'Die Verteilung der Infektionskrankheiten auf Stadt und Land', in *Centralblatt für allgemeine Gesundheitspflege*, vol. 25, 1906

Rothenbacher, F., 'Soziale Ungleichheit des Wohnens in Deutschland im

Bibliography

späten 19. und frühen 20. Jahrhundert', Universität Mannheim 1985 (SFB 3, Arbeitspapier 169, duplicated MS)

——, 'Die Entwicklung der Gesundheitsverhältnisse in Deutschland seit der Industrialisierung', in E. Wiegand and W. Zapf (eds), *Wandel der Lebensbedingungen in Deutschland. Wohlfahrtsentwicklung seit der Industrialisierung*, Frankfurt a.M./New York, 1982

Rothschuh, K.E., *Naturheilbewegung, Reformbewegung, Alternativbewegung*, Stuttgart, 1983

Rott, F., 'Der Rückgang der Säuglingssterblichkeit', in A. Grotjahn (ed.), *Ergebnisse der sozialen Hygiene und Gesundheitsfürsorge*, vol. 1, Leipzig, 1929

Rühle, O., *Illustrierte Kultur- und Sittengeschichte des Proletariats*, vol. 1, Berlin, 1930

Sachße, C., and F. Tennstedt (eds), *Soziale Sicherheit und soziale Disziplinierung. Beiträge zu einer historischen Theorie der Sozialpolitik*, Frankfurt, 1986

Salomon, 'Beseitigung der Abwässer und Abfallstoffe. Reinhaltung der Wasserläufe', in O. Rapmund (ed.), *Das Preußische Medizinal — und Gesundheitswesen in den Jahren 1883–1908*, Berlin, 1908

Sarfatti-Larson, M., *The Rise of Professionalism. A Sociological Analysis*, Berkeley etc., 1977

Schenda, R., 'Das Verhalten der Patienten im Schnittpunkt professionalisierter und naiver Gesundheitsversorgung', in M. Blohmke et al. (eds), *Handbuch der Sozialmedizin*, vol. 3, Stuttgart, 1976

Schmid, J., *Einführung in die Bevölkerungssoziologie*, Reinbek, 1976

Schoenwald, R.L., 'Training Urban Man. A Hypothesis about the Sanitary Movement', in H.J. Dyos and M. Wolff (eds), *The Victorian City: Images and Realities*, vol. 2, London/Boston, 1973

Schröder, W.H., *Arbeitergeschichte und Arbeiterbewegung. Industriearbeit und Organisationsverhalten im 19. und frühen 20. Jahrhundert*, Frankfurt a.M./New York, 1978

Schwabe, K.-H., 'Rassenbiologische Erhebungen in Hennickendorf, einem Dorfe der Mark Brandenburg', in *Archiv für Rassen- und Gesellschaftsbiologie einschl. Rassen- und Gesellschaftshygiene*, vol. 35, 1941

Schwartz, F.W., 'Medizinische Versorgung versus Ernährung — Erklärungskonzepte fuïr die historische Zunahme der Lebenserwartung. Kritische Anmerkungen zur historischen Medizinkritik von Th. McKeown', in *Medizin–Mensch–Gesellschaft*, vol. 9, 1984

Scidlmayer, H., *Geburtenzahl, Säuglingssterblichkeit und Stillung in München in den letzten 50 Jahren*, Munich, 1937

Seiffert, G., 'Das Nichtstillen in Bayern, seine Ursachen und seine Bekämpfung', in *Münchener Medizinische Wochenschrift*, vol. 77, 1930, pt 28

Shorter, E., *Bedside Manners: The Troubled History of Doctors and Patients*, New York, 1985

——, *A History of Women's Bodies*, New York, 1982

Bibliography

——, *The Making of the Modern Family*, New York, 1975
Seutemann, K., *Kindersterblichkeit sozialer Bevölkerungsgruppen insbesondere im preußischen Staate und seinen Provinzen*, Tübingen, 1894
Simson, J. von, 'Kanalisation und Städtehygiene im 19. Jahrhundert', Phil. Diss., Technische Universität Berlin, 1980
Smith, F.B., *The People's Health 1830–1910* London, 1979
Spree, R., 'Veränderungen des Todesursachen-Panoramas und sozio-ökonomischer Wandel — Eine Fallstudie zum "Epidemiologischen Übergang") in G. Gäfgen (ed.), *Ökonomie des Gesundheitswesens*, Berlin 1986 (*Schriften des Vereins für Sozialpolitik*; forthcoming)
——, 'Kurpfuscherei-Bekämpfung und ihre sozialen Funktionen während des 19. und zu Beginn des 20. Jahrhunderts', paper presented to the conference on 'Medizin und sozialer Wandel', ZiF der Universität Bielefeld. 22–24 May 1985 (duplicated MS)
—— et al., 'Ökonomischer Zwang oder schichttypischer Lebensstil? Muster der Einkommensaufbringung und -verwendung vor und nach dem Ersten Weltkrieg', in H. Thomas and F. Elstermann (eds), *Bildung und Beruf. Soziale und ökonomische Aspekte*, Berlin etc., 1985
——, 'Modernisierung des Konsumverhaltens deutscher Mittel- und Unterschichten während der Zwischenkriegszeit', in *Zeitschrift für Soziologie*, 14, 1985, pt 5
——, 'The German Petite Bourgeoisie and the Decline of Fertility: Some Statistical Evidence from the Late-19th and Early-20th Centuries', in *Historical Social Research — Quantum Information*, pt 22, 1982
——, 'Zu den Veränderungen der Volksgesundheit zwischen 1870 und 1913 und ihren Determination in Deutschland (vor allem in Preußen)', in W. Conze and U. Engelhardt (eds), *Arbeiterexistenz im 19. Jahrhundert*, Stuttgart, 1981
——, 'Angestellte als Modernisierungsagenten: Indikatoren und Thesen zum reproduktiven Verhalten von Angestellten im späten 19. und frühen 20. Jahrhundert', in J. Kocka (ed.), *Angestellte Mittelschichten im 19. und 20. Jahrhundert im europäischen Vergleich*, Göttingen, 1981
——, 'The Impact of Professionalization of Physicians on Social Change in Germany during the Late-19th and Early-20th Centuries', in *Historical Social Research — Quantum Information*, pt 15, 1980
——, 'Die Entwicklung der differentiellen Säuglingssterblichkeit in Deutschland seit der Mitte des 19. Jahrhunderts (Ein Versuch zur Mentalitätsgeschichte)', in A.E. Imhof (ed.), *Mensch und Gesundheit in der Geschichte*, Husum, 1980
——, 'Zur Bedeutung des Gesundheitswesens für die Entwicklung der Lebenschancen der deutschen Bevölkerung zwischen 1870 und 1913', in F. Blaich (ed.), *Staatliche Umverteilungspolitik in historischer Perspektive*, Berlin, 1980 (*Schriften des Vereins für Sozialpolitik*, N.F., vol. 109)
——, 'Strukturierte soziale Ungleichheit im Reproduktionsbereich. Zur historischen Analyse ihrer Erscheinungsformen in Deutschland 1870 bis

1913', in J. Bergman et al. (eds), *Geschichte als politische Wissenschaft*, Stuttgart, 1979

Statistisches Jahrbuch für das Deutsche Reich, Jg. 38, 1919

Stearns, P.N., 'The Unskilled and Industrialization. A Transformation of Consciousness', in *Archiv für Sozialgeschichte*, vol. 16, 1976

——, *Lives of Labour. Work in a Maturing Industrial Society*, London, 1975

Stockwell, E.G., 'Infant Mortality and Socio-Economic Status: A Changing Relationship', in *Milbank Memorial Fund Quarterly*, vol. 40, 1962

Stürzbecher, M., 'Die medizinische Versorgung und die Entstehung der Gesundheitsfürsorge zu Beginn des 20. Jahrhunderts in Deutschland', in G. Mann and R. Winau (eds), *Medizin, Naturwissenschaft, Technik und das Zweite Kaiserreich*, Göttingen, 1977

——, 'Aus der Diskussion über das "Klassenlose Krankenhaus" in Alt-Berlin', in *Berliner Ärzteblatt*, vol. 85, 1972, pt 10

——, 'Die Bekämpfung des Geburtenrückganges und der Säuglingssterblichkeit im Spiegel der Reichstagsdebatten 1900–1930. Ein Beitrag zur Geschichte der Bevölkerungspolitik', Phil. Diss., Freie Universität Berlin, 1954

Tennstedt, F., *Vom Proleten zum Industriearbeiter. Arbeiterbewegung und Sozialpolitik in Deutschland 1800 bis 1914*, Cologne, 1983

——, *Sozialgeschichte der Sozialpolitik in Deutschland. Vom 18. Jahrhundert bis zum Ersten Weltkrieg*, Göttingen, 1981

——, 'Sozialgeschichte der Sozialversicherung', in M. Blohmke et al. (eds), *Handbuch der Sozialmedizin*, vol. 3, Stuttgart, 1976

Teuteberg, H.J. (ed.), *Homo Habitans. Zur Sozialgeschichte des ländlichen und städtischen Wohnens in der Neuzeit*, Münster, 1985

—— and C. Wischermann (eds), *Wohnalltag in Deutschland 1850–1914. Bilder–Daten–Dokumente*, Münster, 1985

——, 'Food Consumption in Germany since the Beginning of Industrialization: A Quantitative Longitudinal Approach', in H. Baudet and H. van der Meulen (eds), *Consumer Behaviour and Economic Growth in the Modern Economy*, London/Canberra, 1982

——, 'Wie ernährten sich Arbeiter im Kaiserreich?', in W. Conze and U. Engelhardt (eds), *Arbeiterexistenz im 19. Jahrhundert*, Stuttgart, 1981

——, 'Der Verzehr von Nahrungsmitteln in Deutschland pro Kopf und Jahr seit Beginn der Industrialisierung (1850–1975). Versuch einer quantitativen Langzeitanalyse', in *Archiv für Sozialgeschichte*, vol. 19, 1979

—— and A. Bernhard, 'Wandel der Kindernahrung in der Zeit der Industrialisierung', in J. Reulecke and W. Weber (eds), *Fabrik–Familie–Feierabend. Beiträge zur Sozialgeschichte des Alltags*, Wuppertal, 1978

——, 'Die Nahrung der sozialen Unterschichten im späten 19. Jahrhundert', in E. Heischkel-Artelt (ed.), *Ernährung und Ernährungslehre im 19. Jahrhundert. Vorträge eines Symposiums am 5. u. 6. Januar 1973 in Frankfurt/Main*, Göttingen, 1976

——, 'Studien zur Volksernährung unter sozial- und wirtschaftsgeschichtlichen Aspekten, in idem and G. Wiegelmann, *Der Wandel der Nahrungsgewohnheiten unter dem Einfluß der Industrialisierung*, Göttingen 1972

Titze, H., 'Enrolment Expansion and Academic Overcrowding in Germany', in K.H. Jarausch (ed.), *The Transformation of Higher Learning 1860–1930: Expansion, Diversification, Social Opening and Professionalization in England, Germany, Russia and the United States*, Stuttgart, 1983

——, 'Überfüllungskrisen in akademischen Karrieren: eine Zyklustheorie', in *Zeitschrift für Pädagogik*, vol. 27, 1981, pt 2

Triebel, A., 'Consumption Differentials and War Economy in Germany', in J. Winter and R. Wall (eds), *The Upheaval of War: Family, Work and Welfare in Europe 1914–1918*, Cambridge, 1986

—— and C. Conrad, 'Family Budgets as Sources for Comparative Social History: Western Europe — U.S.A. 1889–1937, in *Historical Social Research — Quantum Information*, pt 35, 1985

——, 'Differential Consumption in Historical Perspective', in *Historical Social Research — Quantum Information*, pt 17, 1981

——, 'Lebensstandarddebatten in der modernen Sozialgeschichtsschreibung. Ein Literaturbericht', Universität Bielefeld, 1977 (unpubl. MS)

Tugendreich, G., 'Der Einfluß der sozialen Lage auf Krankheit und Sterblichkeit des Kindes', in M. Mosse and G. Tugendreich (eds), *Krankheit und soziale Lage*, Munich, 1913

Tutzke, D., 'Der Einfluß der Hygiene und Bakteriologie auf die Medizinalverwaltung in Deutschland vor 1945', in *Zeitschrift für die gesamte Hygiene*, vol. 23, 1977

United Nations, 'Foetal, Infant and Early Childhood Mortality. II: Biological, Social and Economic Factors', in *Population Studies*, vol. 13, 1954

Unschuld, P.U., 'Professionalisierung und ihre Folgen', in H. Schipperges et al. (eds), *Krankheit, Heilkunst, Heilung*, Freiburg i. Br./Munich, 1978

Veröffentlichungen des Kaiserlichen Gesundheitsamtes, vol. 1, Berlin, 1877

Vincent, C.E., 'Trends in Infant Care Ideas', in *Child Development*, vol. 22, 1951, pt 3

Weber, M., *Wirtschaft und Gesellschaft. Grundriß der verstehenden Soziologie*, 5th rev. edn., Tübingen, 1972

Weinberg, W., 'Die Tuberkulose in Stuttgart 1873–1902', in *Medicinisches Correspondenz-Blatt des württembergischen ärztlichen Landesvereins*, vol. 76, 1906

Weindling, P., 'The Medical Profession, Social Hygiene and the Birthrate in Germany 1914–1918', in J. Winter and R. Wall (eds), *The Upheaval of War. Family, Work and Welfare in Europe 1914–1918*, Cambridge, 1986

——, 'The Politics of Hygiene in Imperial Germany', paper presented to the conference on 'Medizin und Sozialer Wandel', ZiF der Universität Bielefeld, 22–24 May 1985 (duplicated MS).

—— (ed.), *The Social History of Occupational Health*, London etc., 1985

Westergaard, H., *Die Lehre von der Mortalität und Morbilität*, 2nd edn., Jena, 1901

Bibliography

Weyl, T., 'Assanierung', in idem (ed.), *Soziale Hygiene*, Jena, 1904 (*Handbuch der Hygiene*, 4th suppl. vol.)

Willie, C.V., 'A Research Note on the Changing Association between Infant Mortality and Socio-Economic Status', in *Social Forces*, vol. 37, 1958/9

Windolf, P. and H.-W. Hohn, *Arbeitsmarktchancen in der Krise. Betriebliche Rekrutierung und soziale Schließung*, Frankfurt a.M./New York, 1984

Wischermann, C., *Wohnen in Hamburg vor dem Ersten Weltkrieg*, Münster, 1983

——, 'Wohnungsnot und Städtewachstum', in W. Conze and U. Engelhardt (eds), *Arbeiter im Industrialisierungsprozeß. Herkunft, Lage und Verhalten*, Stuttgart, 1979

Wolf, J.H., 'Ausstattung und Einrichtung des Krankenhauses in Deutschland 1870–1900', in *Studien zur Krankenhausgeschichte im 19. Jahrhundert im Hinblick auf die Entwicklung in Deutschland*, Göttingen, 1976

Woods, R., and J. Woodward (eds), *Urban Disease and Mortality in Nineteenth-Century England*, London/New York, 1984

Woodward, J., and D. Richards (eds), *Health Care and Popular Medicine in Nineteenth-Century England: Essays in the History of Medicine*, London, 1977

Würzburg, A., 'Über den Einfluß des Alters und des Geschlechts auf die Sterblichkeit an Lungenschwindsucht', in *Mitteilungen aus dem Kaiserlichen Gesundheitsamte*, vol. 2, Berlin, 1884

Zentralverband für Parität der Heilmethoden (eds), *Schriften über Wesen und Bedeutung der Kurierfreiheit*, 1st series, pts 1–6, Berlin, 1911

Index

Aachen, 128
acquisition classes, 13, 15, 18f., 50, 186, 188
alcoholism, 180
Allenstein, 128
anaesthetics, 173
Annales, 4
antisepsis, 107, 119, 173
apothecaries, 161
Arnsberg, 34, 38, 39, 113, 128
artificial feeding, 59, 149
asepsis, 119, 173
Augsburg, 115
Aurich, 128

Bacteriological Research Institutes, 126
bacteriology, 107, 119, 121f., 124, 131, 173
Baden, 161
barger-surgeons, 160, 173
barbers, 160
Barmen, 74, 76, 78
Berlin, 34, 61f., 73, 75, 113, 128, 138–43, 166f., 187
Berlin Medical Society, 166
birth control, 83f., 92f., 100, 102, 146
 see also family planning
birth-rate decline
 harbingers of, 89–91, 94, 101
 social differentials of, 84–95
Black Report, 1
Böckh, R., 73
Boetticher, von, 171, 172
Borscheid, P., 50
bourgeoisie, 164
breast-feeding, 59, 149, 196–202
 campaign for, 72, 75, 77
 father's occupation and, 78–80, 202
 income and, 78–80, 197f., 201
 mothers' occupation and, 76–8, 199
 regional variations in, 74–9, 197f., 201
Bremen, 51
Breslau, 128
Britain, 162

 see also England
Bromberg, 128
Bronfenbrenner, U., 57

calorie consumption, 147
cancer, 45, 49
capitalism, organised, 179
Castell, Gräfin zu, *see* Nell, Adelheid von
cereal prices, 147
child nutrition, 59, 107, 188f.
children per marriage, number of, 84–95, 203–13
 community size and, 86, 92, 205
 father's occupation and, 85–95, 203–13
 rural/urban differentials of, 86, 204
civil service, 93
class formation, 3, 7f., 12f., 15, 17–19, 51, 58, 63, 99, 169, 174, 179, 183, 185
class situation, 13f., 16, 153, 185
classes, various social, *see* social inequality
'Codes of Professional Conduct', 168
Cologne, 128
consumption, per capita, 146f.
Conze, W., 23
croup, 123

Danzig, 128
death, causes of, 32–4, 40f., 43–6, 123
 according to age group, 44–6, 48–50
 pattern of, 48
 regional variations of, 46, 48f.
Decree on Medicine (*Medizinalordnung*), 161
demographic transition, 92
Dickler, R., 107, 147
diet, 58f., 71–80, 106, 130, 132, 143f., 146, 148f.
differential association, 14, 16f., 187
diphtheria, 123f.
disability insurance funds, expenditures on TB treatment, 119f.

241

Index

see also tuberculosis
diseases
  chronic, 49–54
  infectious, 30–2, 40–2, 48f., 123, 127, 130f., 133, 138, 141, 147f., 151f.
  pulmonary, 41–6
disinfection, 125f., 132
dispensaries for infants and mothers, 75
doctors, 8, 17, 31, 75, 106f., 111, 126, 130–2, 151, 158–183
  incomes of, 167
  labour market for, 168
  number of, 110, 113–15, 150, 168
  per head of population, 112, 148
  privileges of, 164, 166, 170f.
  social regulation of work, 171
  social status of, 160–9
Dortmund, 34
drainage, 186
Düsseldorf, 34, 37–9, 76, 128

ecological approach, 51, 60
ecology of human development, 57
Edelstein, W., 9
educated classes, 161, 164
education system, 97, 99
enforced socialisation, 4, 178f., 181–3, 187
England, 107
  see also Britain
epidemics, 30f., 126, 129, 131, 138
Erfurt, 128
Essen, 34
Ethical Committees (*Ehrenräte*), 167f.
expert knowledge, 160f., 164
experts, status of, 167

factory rules, 181
family planning, 83, 100, 102, 180, 183
  see also birth control
family size models, 58f., 88–90
fecundity, see fertility
Federation of Medical Associations (*Ärztevereinsbund*), 168
Ferber, C. von, 178
fertility, 87, 90–4, 182
  decline of, 87–95
  timing and, 87–95
Fischer, A., 24
food hygiene policy, 124
food research institutes, 124
food supplies, 152

Frankfurt am Main, 34, 60f.
Frankfurt an der Oder, 113, 128

gastro-intestinal infections, 43–5, 148
Geldern, 74
German Working Men's Brotherhood (*Grundstatuten der Deutscher Arbeiter-Verbrüderung*), 27
Giddens, A., 13
'great killers', 41–4, 151
Grevenbroich, 74
Gumbinnen, 34, 37, 128

Haines, M., 93f.
Hamburg, 121–3
Hanover, 74, 76–80, 128
healers, 110f.
  see also lay healers
health
  attitudes towards, 178, 188
  concept of, 27
  expropriation of, 165
  indicators of, 26, 28–35
  inequalities in, 1, 4, 16
  perceptions of, 174
health care, 110, 113, 162–5, 179, 183
health education, 151
Health Reports, 125f., 129, 137
health sector, 99, 105–11, 114, 129, 131, 167, 187
  expansion of, 150, 153
  quality of, 119, 121
health service, 144, 181
health services, market for, 158, 169–77, 181–3
health standards, 106, 186, 188
Helberger, C., 28
Hildesheim, 128
history of medicine, see medicine
Hobrecht, J., 141
Hoffman, W.G., 147
hospital care, days spent in, 47
  quality of, 116–18
  regional variations, 128f.
hospital service, expansion of, 114, 168
hospital treatment, 98, 117, 129, 173
hospitals
  beds in, 114f., 127, 148, 150
  doctors in, 114f., 118
  general, 114, 117, 127
  number of, 150
  patients in, 217
household remedies, 111
housing

242

Index

overcrowded, 61f., 142
quality of, 58f., 61f., 123, 142f., 149
shortage of, 106, 123
housing welfare, 180
Huerkamp, C., 160
hygiene, 59, 123, 132
  domestic, 75, 81, 122, 133, 152, 186
  personal, 107
  public, 130f.
  racial, 182
  social, 122
  standards of, 180
  urban, 75

illegitimate children, 66, 78
illness, attitudes towards, 178
Imperial Food Act (*Reichsnahrungsgesetz*), 124
Imperial Health Office (*Kaiserliches Gesundheitsamst*), 30, 31, 41, 135
income
  average, 145
  distribution of, 146, 148
  real, 106
  see also wages, real
industrialisation, 2, 4, 106, 174
infant care, 5, 57
infant health, 3
infant mortality, 7, 35f., 38, 43, 55–84, 90, 92, 94–6, 101, 148, 152, 180, 182, 186, 188
  conceptual framework of, 56–9
  determinants of, 56–9, 62
  among domestics/household servants, 65–71
  neo-natal, 69–71
  post-natal, 69–71
  among public officials, 65–71
  rates of, 35–7, 60–80, 191–6, 198
  among self-employed, 65–71
  among skilled workers, 65–71
  surveys on, 60, 73–80
  among unskilled workers, 65–71
  among white-collar workers, 65–71
infrastructure, 108, 177, 186, 187
  expansion of, 144
  facilities, 99, 142
  health-related, 18, 105f., 109, 131, 143f., 148, 151f., 180–3
  hidden curriculum of, 181
  innovations in, 131

Kassel, 128
Knodel, J., 91, 92

Koblenz, 128
Koch, R., 121, 123, 125
Kocka, J., 24
Königsberg, 34, 37, 128
Köslin, 113, 128

labour movement, 100, 152, 169, 179, 182, 185, 188
lay healers, 110f., 114, 161f., 165f., 171f., 174f.
leach-pit system, 141, 142
Lee, R.W., 107f.
legislation on medicine, *see* medicine
Leipzig, 60–2
Liegnitz, 128
life chances, 96–101, 105, 143, 153, 180, 183, 185
life expectancy, 23, 36, 106, 144
life style, 6, 14, 16f., 96, 101, 132, 174, 182
  changes in, 169
  rationalisation of, 93, 180f.
  urban industrial, 148
Linden, 74, 76f., 79f.
Löffler, F., 124
Lower Saxony, 84
Lüneburg, 128

McKeown, T., 8, 106, 107
Magdeburg, 128
Marienwerder, 128
market capacity, 14f., 16, 18f., 50, 54, 58f., 63, 96, 98f., 105, 143, 183, 185–8
market conditions, 167
market forces, 105
market situation, causal components of, 81, 96
Max Planck Institute of Educational Research, 5, 9
measurement, problems of, 26
mcat, 146f.
medical
  assistants, 162
  associations, 168f., 171, 175
  care, 148
    level of, 112, 114
  culture, 180
  monopoly, 171, 173, 178
  officers, 113f.
  policing, 161, 164
  profession, 3, 17f., 157, 167f., 174
    autonomy of, 157f., 160f., 163
    ethic, 157, 169

243

medicine in, 111
  authority of, 172
  monopoly of, 158, 162
  qualifications, 100
  saturation of, 175
  status, 153
  training, 174
  see also professionalisation
  reforms, 164f., 169
  research, 125, 158, 160
  science, 107, 127, 131, 150f., 163, 167f., 173, 182
  screening, 180
  services, quality of, 186
  students, number of, 168, 175
  technology, 158, 168, 173
  therapy, 124, 171f.
  training, 158, 162f., 169
Medical Report, 172
medicalisation, 159, 176f., 179, 182f., 188
medicine
  history of, 124
  legislation on, 124
  social history of, 2–4
Meerwarth, R., 91
mentalities, 3f., 94f., 174, 181–3, 187f.
  rationalist, 95
  see also rationalist value-system
Merseburg, 128
miasmas, 131
microbiology, 173
midwives, 161f.
Minden, 128
modernisation, 5f., 96, 98, 153
Mönchengladbach, 79
mortality, 106f., 128
  decline in, 8
mortality rate
  average, 32, 35–7, 47f., 191f., 217
  and water supply system, 143
mortality rates, 52, 107, 128, 130, 132, 141f., 145, 148
  and specific age groups, 37–40, 191f.
mothers
  and factory work, 78, 81
  level of employment of, 76–80
  unmarried, 76f.
Munich, 60, 62, 137
Münster, 128

natural healing, 172f.
  associations for the cultivation of, 173

Nell, Adelheid von (Gräfin zu Castell), 84, 93, 101
neo-natal infant mortality, *see* infant mortality
Neuß, 74
nurses, 118, 126, 162, 173
nutrition methods, 58, 188

obstetrics, 173
Occupational Census, 59
occupational groups, 65–71, 78–80, 84–95
occupational health, 25, 34f.
occupational status, 63
Oppeln, 116, 128
Osnabrück, 128
Ottmüller, U., 9

paediatrics, 5
parity-dependent control, 92
Parry, J., 17
patients, 132
'people's health' (*Volksgesundheit*), 23, 25f., 30, 32, 34f., 105f., 111, 133
  changing trends in, 47–54
Pettenkofer, M. von, 132, 137
Pflanz, M., 151
plague, 132
poisonous vapours, 131
political involvement, 100
poorhouse, 129
population policy, 180
Posen, 128
post-natal infant mortality, *see* infant mortality
potatoes, 146f.
Potsdam, 128
poverty syndrome, 51, 75, 81, 82
Preston, S.H., 107
Preußische Statistik, 33, 59
Prinzing, F., 34
professionalisation, 3, 17, 18, 114, 168–70, 179, 181–3
  concept of, 157–9, 162, 166
  see also medical
protein deficit, 145
Prussia, 33, 36–40, 42, 46, 48, 52, 64, 66, 70, 74, 108, 113, 122, 125, 127, 133–6, 148, 161f.
  cities in, 39
  Eastern provinces of, 147
Prussian Criminal Code, 166
Prussian Medical Administration, 176
public health, 108, 121f., 125, 127,

244

Index

132, 151, 153, 180
laboratory, 125
officers, 75, 161
standards, 136, 144
'Public Health Campaign' (*Kampf der Hygieniker*), 137
pulmonary diseases, *see* diseases

quackery, fight against, 175f.
quacks, 110, 162, 165–7, 171
  number of, 113
qualification crisis, 97
quarantine, 107

rationalist value-system, 6, 100, 177
  see also mentalities
regional inequality, 46, 48f., 71–80, 110, 128f., 133–9, 191, 197f., 201, 214f., 217–21
Reichstag, 166, 171
reproductive behaviour, 5f., 83, 92–4, 101
Rheydt, 74
Ritter, G.A., 24
Rott, F., 123
Rühle, O., 25

sanatoria, 119–23
Saxony, 59, 70
Schleswig, 128
Schomerus, H., 50
sewerage systems, 75, 133, 152, 180
  by town size, 136
sickness, sliding scale of, 28
sickness insurance, 2f., 27, 29, 115, 128, 150, 168f., 172, 176, 181
Sickness Insurance Act, 97, 169, 171, 178, 180f.
sickness insurance funds, members of, 29f., 47, 115f., 129, 216
Sigmaringen, 128
Silesia, 116
smallpox vaccine, 132
Smith, F.B., 2
social
  attitudes, 105
  change, 181, 183
  decline, collective, 186
  homogenisation, 182
  indicators, 117
  inequality, 5, 15, 56f., 62, 91, 101, 105, 110, 129, 153, 174
    concept of, 11–19, 185
    structures of, 7f., 12, 18f., 54, 82, 95, 108, 112, 162, 179, 182f., 188
  mobility, upward, 101, 163
  policy, 180, 187
  regulation of doctor's work, *see* doctors
  stratification, 2, 5f., 11, 14f., 16, 18f., 34, 63, 96, 153, 174, 187f.
social history of medicine, *see* medicine
social security system, 18, 75, 183, 186f.
soil or ground theory, 132
Sonderweg, 4
Stade, 128
standard of living, 144f.
status groups, 16f., 18, 94, 99
Stearns, P.N., 25
Stettin, 128
Stralsund, 128
street-cleaning, 133, 152, 186
strokes, 43f.
Stuttgart, 53
surgeons, 160–2, 173

Teuteberg, H.J., 146f.
therapeutic chaos, 163
therapeutic medicine, effectiveness, 107, 123–30, 173
Trade Acts (*Gewerbeordnungen*), 110, 161f., 166f., 171
trade union methods, 170
trade unions, 100, 152
Triebel, A., 9
Trier, 128
tuberculin, 122
tuberculosis, 41–5, 48, 52–4, 121, 123, 152, 180, 186
  mortality rate for, 121–3
  number of patients cured of, 119f.
  sanatoria for patients, 121
  therapy for, 119, 123
  tuberculosis bacillus, 121f.
typhoid, 123, 125, 137
  campaign against, 125
  incidence of, 140, 142f., 187
typhus, 122

undernutrition, 145
University Institutes of Hygiene, 126
urban population, 86, 150
urban sanitation, 107, 121, 130, 133, 152, 180, 186
urbanisation, 169, 174
USA, 162

values, patterns of, 182, 187f.
Virchow, R., 141
Volkskrankheiten ('epidemic diseases'), 30
  see also epidemics
Vorwärts, Der, 25

wages, real, 130, 152, 169
Wales, 107
water supply systems, 75, 133, 139–43, 152, 180, 186f.
  by town size, 134f., 218–20

WCs, 141f.
weaning, moment of, 78–80
Weber, M., 3, 13, 16f., 81, 96, 98
welfare systems, 180, 183, 186f.
wells, 137
whooping cough, 122
Wiesbaden, 128
working conditions, 46, 50–2, 100, 186
working days lost, number of, 47

X-rays, 173